Managing perioperative care:
Influences on surgery and nursing

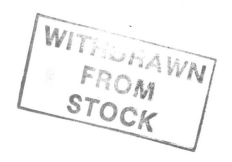

Managing perioperative care:
Influences on surgery and nursing

Marilyn Williams

Quay
Books

Mark Allen
Publishing Ltd

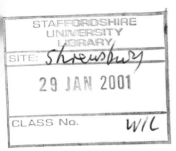
Quay Books Division, Mark Allen Publishing Limited
Jesses Farm, Snow Hill, Dinton, Wiltshire, SP3 5HN

British Library Cataloguing-in-Publication Data
A catalogue record is available for this book

© Mark Allen Publishing Ltd 2000
ISBN 1 85642 092 2

Printed in the UK by Cromwell Press, Trowbridge, Wiltshire

1
Contents

Acknowledgements

This book represents a further demonstration of faith in my abilities by Roswyn Brown and Quay Books. I am deeply grateful for being offered the chance to write it.

In writing this book I have called upon the advice, memories and reminiscences of doctor and nurse colleagues past and present. They have all co-operated fully and generously, giving me their time and answering my persistent and sometimes provocative questions with patience and honesty. I must particularly mention Bernard Williams, a Consultant Neurosurgeon with whom I worked for many years. I interviewed him at some length on 16 June 1995. Within a few weeks of that interview he was injured in a road traffic accident and died on 10 August 1995. Bernard had a profound influence on my career as a theatre sister, I admired him greatly for his immense surgical skill and his unfailing honesty. I am extremely grateful that he was able to contribute to this work.

Marilyn Williams
April, 2000

Foreword

I was delighted to have been asked to write the foreword to Marilyn's latest book. I have long been an admirer of her writings and amusing presentations of papers at conferences.

This latest offering is a well written treatise on many of the issues that are infrequently addressed in relation to perioperative practice; ethics, advocacy, teamwork, dealing with professions, research, humour and recent developments in surgical techniques and day care. In many respects it is a reader or starter book, and certainly the key to developing thinking which enables and develops practitioners.

A book of this nature of necessity travels over a number of different areas of practice; of clinical, educational and managerial practice and adds a portion of audit and research. Indeed, it reflects the all-round approach to perioperative practice required of the competent, well-qualified perioperative nurse today. It was not always so and the massive strides made over recent years, well certainly the years that Marilyn reflects, are sometimes only realised when one looks back. It is said in different ways that one needs to look back before one can look forward and although that is not the entirety of 'reflective practice', it is complimentary to it.

One of the drivers in the National Health Service today is the need to work towards integration and understanding; integration of the various services and between the agencies that provide those services and understanding between professional staff which has been such a positive aspect, tempered only by the shock of the obvious lack of understanding that existed previously. Hopefully, this book will inform the debate and highlight some of the areas of practice that are moving forward apace.

One of the biggest challenges facing perioperative nurses currently is to engage in meaningful dialogue with users of the service so that quality of care can be improved. The term 'users' in this context will certainly include other staff using the facilities but strategies of improvement will be worthless without input from patients. That will be an area of ground-breaking proportions for some and not easy for anyone but it affords great opportunity to take perioperative nursing forward into this century. Marilyn refers to the 'influences on surgery and nursing' as a theme so do take time to reflect on the themes within her excellent book to inform your future.

In case any form of mutual admiration society should be emerging, let me add that there is something missing. That, of course, is you, who choose to read this book. You are the only one who con provide the intelligence to bridge the theory/ reality gap and who can give life to this work. I recommend that you do precisely that.

Libby Campbell OBE, RGN, RM, MSc

April, 2000

Miss EM Campbell is Director of Nursing and Quality at St John's Hospital at Howden and was Chairman of the National Association of Theatre Nurses from 1992 to 1995. She is currently a member of the Editorial Board of the *British Journal of Theatre Nursing*.

Preface

This book is intended to inform and guide the perioperative nurse through many of the issues which influence professional practice today. I use the word 'perioperative' quite deliberately, as 'theatre nursing' carries with it the assumption that only what happens behind closed doors is important. Increasingly, nurses are having to come out from behind those closed doors and broaden their outlook, challenge and change their practice. This book gives an insight into some of the issues which will be part of that broader outlook.

This is not a 'how to do it' book. Learning to be a perioperative nurse is a personal and practical adventure which could not be effectively translated into text. What is offered is information and an exploration of many of the subjects, controversies and debates which impinge on the people delivering care to surgical patients. For qualified nurses on post basic courses, this is one of a few UK texts which address perioperative care. Much of the established perioperative literature is from the United States and, though useful, some of that information may not translate so well into our health care system.

I have drawn extensively on my personal experience as a theatre nurse for over 20 years, as well as my more recent involvement with nurse education. One of the real pleasures of my current post is that I am still able to spend time being involved with students and qualified staff in operating theatres. I remain an active and committed member of the National Association of Theatre Nurses and take a pride in keeping up to date with current issues in perioperative care. I hope that you will enjoy reading this book and go on to enjoy perioperative nursing as much as I did as a practitioner and still do as a teacher.

Marilyn Williams
April, 2000

1

'Another fine mess you've got me into...'

History

When surgeons first began to develop their art, they were condemned as barbarians by their fellow physicians. For many years surgery remained a foul and mysterious occupation. Inevitably, and with some reason connected to the robbing of graves and gruesome dissections which were to contribute to our learning about the physical body and how it worked.

Surgery developed as an offshoot of barbering. The men who cut hair would also pull teeth and lance boils. Little wonder that the high class, educated men who held office as physicians wanted nothing to do with this low life overlap into their territory. A remnant of this division remains in Britain today, with the common title 'Mr' accorded to surgeons, as opposed to 'Doctor' for physicians. Even those we refer to as 'Doctor' in medicine, have stolen this title from the academic world and made it their own, such is the elitism that was once attached to learning, and still is in some circles.

It took many years for surgery to become accepted as a legitimate method for treating disease. Once established in hospitals, surgery remained an exclusively male province in that the only people involved in performing it were doctors and medical students. As surgery became more successful, with the development of antiseptic measures, anaesthesia, and complex instrumentation, skilled help for the surgeon became more important. Medical students continued to play a major part in assisting surgeons, but inevitably moved on to pursue their own careers and so were a constantly changing and inconsistent source of help. Nurses, however, were becoming organised themselves. Recognised training and eventually registration raised the status of nursing and nurses. Here was a constant presence of female servants to the sick and the doctors.

It is not really surprising then that surgeons took nurses into theatre to help them. Here was someone who would do as they were told, learn about the materials required for an operation, prepare them, hand them to the surgeon in the correct sequence, clean up afterwards and look after the patient. And, of course, because this person was female, however good she became at her job, she posed no threat whatever to the eminent surgeon, unlike the upstart medical student who might learn everything the surgeon had to teach, get even better at it, and steal his master's practice! Gender issues in relation to work in the caring professions may not be as obvious today, but they certainly have not gone away (Hugman, 1991).

Nursing in its earliest days of organisation was regarded as a superior form of domestic service, indeed many early recruits came from a background of domestic service, and were supervised by middle class ladies, without actual nursing skills, but who acted as domestic managers and became the matrons who influenced nursing for many years (Dingwall *et al*, 1988). In taking on a domestic service model, nursing from its beginnings was task orientated and female dominated. Just as a middle class woman would expect her servants to do and have done certain things at certain times, so this became the expected role for nurses in hospitals. Remnants of it survive in hospitals to this day, in spite of the nursing process, research-based practice, education for holistic care, and a patient centred philosophy (White, 1985).

So a nursing presence became established in operating theatres. Mackay (1993) graphically and accurately describes theatre nursing, with particular reference to the 'shared intimacy between medical and nursing staff which is seldom experienced in the wards'.

This is certainly true of the present day situation, where close working relationships are often formed in theatre teams (Williams, 1995). Close relationships between doctors and nurses have an historical precedent. McGann (1992) describes the conditions in Glasgow Royal Infirmary at the turn of the last century:

> *Nurses were divided into day and night nurses, one of each class being assigned to each ward, and they worked exclusively for the physician or surgeon of that ward.*

Here is clear evidence of medicine coming to expect and rely on a constant source of care for patients. Although the reliance of one group on the other is clear, the hierarchies of both medicine and nursing suffered from class and gender assumptions as well as conflicts between themselves (Hugman, 1991). Remnants of these assumptions and conflicts are still in evidence, particularly in operating theatre nursing. Medicine is firmly established as a profession, nursing is still striving to become one. Nursing is now a highly organised discipline, developing its own research base and an increasing number of specialities. A dated but still delightful description of theatre teamwork contains the very true observation that:

> *So necessary is teamwork, in the nature of the job, that even individuals who are personally antagonistic often act in concert during the course of surgery.*

Wilson, 1954

The doctor — nurse game

The relationship between nursing and medicine reflects the gender divisions which characterised the early development of both disciplines. The male doctor was educated, authoritative and in control. The first nurses were subservient, dutiful and obedient. Pilliteri and Ackerman (1993) quote Florence Nightingale who when reporting doctors' expectations of nurses as being those of 'devotion and obedience', responded that:

> *This definition would do just as well for a porter. It might even do for a horse.*

The doctor — nurse game still survives in operating theatres, though the acting out of it is sometimes more subtle. Stein *et al* (1990) declare that nurses have stopped playing the game, and become assertive professionals making an equal contribution to care. The author believes that some nurses in the United Kingdom have some way to go yet to be seen in that light. Subservience to medical domination is still alive and well in many operating theatres.

Theatre nursing as a speciality

Theatre nursing is firmly established as a speciality within nursing, and has its own representative body, the National Association of Theatre Nurses (NATN). The Association currently represents nearly half of all of the nurses working in operating theatres in the United Kingdom. It has important European and international connections. From small local beginnings in the 1960s, the national profile of NATN is now such that it is recognised as the 'voice' of theatre nursing in the United Kingdom. The Department of Health, Scottish, Welsh and Northern Ireland offices regularly seek advice and comment from NATN on matters pertaining to operating theatres and practices within them. The Association has also co-operated with the Royal College of Surgeons on various matters, including being involved with training doctors and nurses in minimally invasive surgical techniques.

Today's operating theatre nurse is expected to assume many roles. The expectations that surgeons and anaesthetists have of theatre nurses are more fully explored in *Chapter 3*. At this point, the professional and autonomous roles of theatre nurses will be explored.

Roles, rules and divisions

Operating theatres are staffed by a variety of disciplines, and the person in charge may be from any of the disciplines or be independent of all of them, employed by the hospital or Trust to manage and deliver surgical services. Within this organisation there are nurses, employed to provide a nursing service. The question of whether the work of nurses in operating theatres actually constitutes nursing is contentious. Where nursing takes place in a highly structured and technologically complex environment, it is all too easy to lose the patient in the machinery, and reduce the process to a production line.

The development of new posts in surgery such as 'Surgical assistant' have provided nurses and others with opportunities to develop new roles and skills. In the past, the only person who would have acted as a surgeon's assistant would have been another doctor, usually of a lower rank, or a medical student. Now nurses, operating department assistants (ODAs) and operating department practitioners (ODPs) are being appointed to surgeon's assistant posts, where they take an active part in surgical interventions, under the supervision of the surgeon. Additionally, they may be involved in pre-assessment clinics, pre-operative preparation, and post-operative management, including dealing with pain and wound management. An explanation of the origins of ODAs and ODPs is needed here to clarify their position.

ODAs have been a part of operating theatre staff for many years, sometimes evolving from a theatre porter role, now they are a vital part of the operating team. A City &

Guilds qualification was the first recognition of the importance of the ODAs role, and this has now been replaced by the national vocational qualification (NVQ) of operating department practitioner (ODP). There is much overlap between the roles of ODPs and nurses.

There is some debate as to the legitimacy of surgical assistant roles for nurses, as they seem to be what junior doctors did in the past. An alternative and more positive view is that for a nurse to be involved with the patient from before admission, through surgery and recovery to discharge, reflects a truly holistic nursing role. Some nurses are doing this very successfully in the field of laparoscopic surgery (Williams, 1996). The English National Board (ENB) has validated a post basic qualification for surgeons' assistants, giving further impetus to developing nursing roles into new areas.

The Scope of Professional Practice

This document was issued by the UKCC in 1994. The idea behind it is that nurses may prescribe their own boundaries to practice, in conjunction with their employers. Specific roles and responsibilities are made explicit in job descriptions, so that all parties are aware of what any nurse is capable and competent to undertake.

Previously, certain tasks such as intravenous cannulation and intravenous drug administration were designated as 'extended role' nursing. In order to be able to undertake such tasks, qualified nurses had to undertake further 'training', consisting of a variety of lengths of theoretical input (eg. one or two days), followed by some practical sessions during which the nurse would be expected to attain competence in the task. A written statement of competence would then be issued. As these arrangements were specific not only to tasks, but to hospitals and employers, they were not transferable between jobs.

The UKCC's view is that such arrangements are anti-professional, and demean nursing as a series of tasks, rather than the actions of an holistic and research-based autonomous practitioner, seen to be the nurse of the future. This is a valid view if nurses are to become autonomous professionals in their own right. Doctors and lawyers who are firmly established as professionals do not describe or prescribe their practice in terms of definitive tasks.

Expanding the boundaries of nursing practice emerged at the same time as an increased interest in reducing junior doctors working hours. Maybe this was coincidental. Nurses now have a great deal of freedom of choice in career pathways, some will relish the prospect of developing surgical skills and literally carving out a career as a surgical assistant. Others will wish to retain a more traditional role. There are a variety of other options available. The important issue is that nurses do not become cheap doctors, readily picking up technical duties which the medical profession chooses to discard.

Nursing has already 'sold off' areas of care, such as giving out meals and washing patients, and is still looking for an answer to the question 'what is nursing?' This has even more significance for operating theatre nurses, whose role and presence has been the question of debate for many years.

Preparation, continuing education and training

Preparation

Nurses prepared through Project 2000 and now RN DipHE or RN BSc courses are often not allocated to operating theatres during their course (Matthews, 1995). The reasons for this are varied. Sometimes, there are just too many students in a group, so some go to theatre but not all. It could be and sometimes is argued that current university nursing courses with their focus on health, present an ideological conflict to operating theatre nursing (Matthews, 1995), and indeed, some nurse teachers do not see an allocation to operating theatres as a necessary part of student preparation for practice. The author does not share this view. Baxter (1996) convincingly dismisses Matthews' (1995) arguments, making plain the nursing role and function in operating theatres, by highlighting the similarities with nursing in any other environment.

One dimension of nursing comes into its own in operating theatres — patient advocacy. Where the patient is vulnerable, completely dependent, and unable to speak for himself, the theatre nurse is present to act and speak on his behalf (Marshall, 1994), and this is surely a most compelling reason for a nursing presence in theatres. Others may argue that anyone in theatre may act as the patient's advocate, and this is true, but the only person who is obligated to do so is the nurse.

As well as being the patients' advocate, today's nursing students are encouraged to question and challenge all aspects of practice. Some currently practising nurses are not comfortable with this and use it as an excuse for criticising university training programmes (Williams, 1999).

The evolution of Project 2000 programmes into Registered Nurse, Diploma in Higher Education (RN Dip HE), and Registered Nurse, Bachelor of Science (RN BSc) courses, as well as other academic pathways, has resolved some of the early problems of transferring nursing into higher education. Trusts, universities and the UKCC have collaborated in producing a variety of curricula and awards which are designed to meet the needs of future nurses and their patients. Allocating student nurses to operating theatres for a part of their training is now common practice once again.

Continuing education

All of nurse education is now a part of the university system. The National Boards validate curricula prepared by departments or faculties of nursing, forming a pathway through higher education to diploma and degree qualifications. Several courses are available which are directly concerned with operating theatre nursing. These initiatives, combined with the now mandatory requirement to maintain a minimal level of continuing education, provide opportunities for theatre nurses to develop their knowledge, enabling the delivery of well-informed care to their patients.

As a part of continuity of care, the theatre nurse takes over where the ward nurse leaves off, assuming responsibility for the nursing care of that patient during the time spent in the operating department. When viewed in this way, operating theatre nursing can clearly be seen to be a vital and necessary part of care. The myth that theatre nurses just look after surgeons and instruments is just that — a myth (McGee, 1994). Specialist qualifications in operating theatre practice, leading to diplomas and degrees reflect the continued importance of this speciality.

Training

The difference between education and training is becoming increasingly blurred. Each has always overlapped the other to some extent. Dictionary definitions usually include 'knowledge' under education, and 'skill' under training. Education may also be interpreted as including an implied level of accountability for the use of knowledge.

Vocational qualifications, which in the past may have been seen as purely skills based, now have a well established place in the higher education system. In operating theatre practice, vocational qualifications are available for all grades of staff. In the future, all theatre staff may well hold some sort of qualification for whatever post they hold. Pathways for progression are already in place for theatre staff to move through training and educational systems, to many types of qualification.

Conclusion

After men began cutting up their fellows, the realisation that help was needed to do this came quickly. First the apprentice surgeon, then the compliant nurse, followed the surgical pioneers into theatre. Those compliant nurses eventually became organised and assertive in their own right, forming the National Association of Theatre Nurses in 1964. The nurse first went into theatre to look after the patient, and is still doing that today.

From the earliest days of barber surgeons, through the development of antiseptic surgery, anaesthesia, gender conflicts and world wars, today's operating theatres are now areas of skilful practice for many occupations and professions. The need for these groups to work together in a co-operative, collaborative manner, in the name of high quality patient care, has never been more urgent. The policy imperatives of clinical governance and evidence-based healthcare are already in place. We need now to ensure that these are coupled with the capturing of hearts and minds of a committed multidisciplinary healthcare workforce.

References

Baxter B (1996) The role of the nurse in theatre. A reply. *Br J Theatre Nurs* **5**(11): 5–6

Dingwall R, Rafferty A, Webster C (1988) *An Introduction to the Social History of Nursing*. Routledge, London

Hugman R (1991) *Power in Caring Professions*. MacMillan, Basingstoke

Mackay L (1993) *Conflicts in Care, Medicine and Nursing*. Chapman & Hall, London

McGann S (1992) *Battle of the Nurses*. Scutari Press, London

McGee P (1994) Rediscovering theatre nursing. *Br J Theatre Nurs* **4**(3): 8–10

Marshall C (1994) The concept of advocacy. *Br J Theatre Nurs* **4**(2): 11–13

Matthews E (1995) Where have all the student nurses gone? *Br J Theatre Nurs* **5**(9): 18–21

Pilliteri A, Ackerman M (1993) The 'Doctor-Nurse' Game: A Comparison of 100 Years — 1888–1990. *Nurs Outlook* **41**: 113–116

Stein L, Watts D, Howell T (1990) The Doctor-Nurse Game Revisited. *Nurs Outlook* Nov/Dec: 264–268

White R (ed) (1985) *Political Issues in Nursing*, Volume 1. John Wiley & Sons, Chichester

Williams M (1995) Challenging nursing myths and traditions. *Br J Theatre Nurs* **5**(9): 8–11

Williams M (1996) The expanding role of the nurse in laparoscopic surgery. *Br J Theatre Nurs* **6**(4): 34–35

Williams M (1999) Nurse education has had a bad press. *Br J Theatre Nurs* **9**(6): 245

Wilson R (1954) *Teamwork in the Operating Room*. Human Organisation, Winter: 9–14

United Kingdom Central Council for Nursing, Midwifery and Health Visiting (1994) *The Scope of Professional Practice.* UKCC, London

2

Nursing knowledge and specialisation

Nurses gain their knowledge from many sources, including theoretical instruction and from practice. It is generally accepted that the majority of learning takes place in practice, both before and after gaining first registration (Williams, 1996a). Conway's (1995) study of the evolution of expert nursing knowledge reveals the importance of organisational culture in promoting or hindering the acquisition of various types of knowledge, skills and attitudes.

Operating theatres tend to generate microcultures, even within large operating suites. In this sense, work may take on a 'social' context which is known to influence the process of learning (Hart and Rotem, 1995). Working in such a culture could lead to the development of significant expertise for nurses, who have an opportunity to become extremely skilled in one type of surgery. Alternatively, isolation from the mainstream of nursing and from peers may produce a limited and inhibited nurse who is only able to function within clearly prescribed boundaries.

Valuing nursing

Attitudes to nursing knowledge are indicative of the value attached to nursing itself and as much of the work of nursing is invisible, such a value may be difficult to determine (Neubaur, 1995). Delamothe (1988) saw this as a problem of stereotyping, stemming from the historical linking of nursing with women's work in general, and the lowly values traditionally associated with this. Having changed the preparation of nurses from an apprenticeship system to a university academic system, nursing and the knowledge embedded in its practice may in future assume a higher value. Lawson (1996) roundly condemns the academic route to nursing registration, though bases some of her criticism on erroneous information regarding entry requirements. The thrust of her argument appears to be that nursing does not require a high level of intellect or knowledge, so a few well educated nurses to lead a large 'infantry' (her word) of hands on carers will solve all nursing's problems. In direct contrast to this, Castledine (1997) emphasises the need for recognition of clinical career structures to keep skilled nurses in contact with patients, rather than the current situation where promotion almost always leads to managerial or other non clinical posts. He declares that:

> *Careers in clinical nursing should be soundly based on post registration education and experience.*

This is a view much more in touch with reality than Lawson's.

Glen (1995) acknowledges the problems implicit in placing nurse education in the university system, and advocates closer collaboration in research between educationalists and practitioners. She sees this as an answer to the theory practice gap. Apart from closing the theory practice gap, Glen (1995) goes further in her argument in favour of nursing's place in higher education:

> *The process should promise a freeing of the mind, but also beyond, to bring about a new level of self empowerment in the individual student. In essence it should contain an emancipatory element.*

While admiring and agreeing wholeheartedly with these sentiments, this author's personal experience of current operating theatre nurses is that many of them are not ready for such freedoms. They are caught up in a politically manipulated system which rewards quantity above all, expects more for the same or less resources, and suppresses any challenge to medical domination.

Nursing knowledge

Much of the knowledge which theatre nurses have is demonstrated in hands on skills with instruments and techniques. Learning such skills is a very individual process, and the subject of a number of theories (Steinaker and Bell, 1979; Rogers, 1983; Kolb, 1984). In addition, Langstaff and Gray (1997) see a danger in nurses 'becoming locked into one area of expertise' and call for a flexible approach to role development in order to avoid the risk of 'burnout from long service in a stressful environment'. This is certainly a possibility in operating theatres.

A further consideration is the interchangeability of doctors and nurses, arising from a radical overhaul of the skill mix in both primary and hospital care. A major report in which the literature on skill mix was reviewed suggests that:

> *Between 30 and 70 per cent of the tasks performed by doctors could be carried out by nurses, and it is shown that hundreds of millions of pounds might be saved if skill mix could be altered in this way.*

> Richardson and Maynard, 1995

If this is indeed a valid conclusion, developing theatre nurses skills from handing the tools to doing the surgery seems to be a logical and acceptable step. It is already a fact for some nurses in the UK (Erikson, 1996). This logical progression in skills represents a significant transfer of knowledge for nurses, whose preparation and training are focused toward caring holistically and meeting individual needs, whereas the doctor concentrates on disease processes, diagnosis and treatments.

The knowledge bases from which doctors and nurses work are radically different, with nursing still striving to establish its own research base. Medicine has the distinct advantage of basing diagnosis and treatment on strictly controlled research and randomised trials, where an outcome can be proven beyond doubt. Just because nursing is not always able to act from a basis of scientific certainty, it does not mean that nursing knowledge is any less worthy. Nursing is the service closest to the patient, and high quality care is often invisible, being appreciated in many intangible ways such as the relief of pain and prevention of complications (Neubaur, 1995).

Specialisation

Much of the knowledge embedded in theatre nursing practice is procedural, operational and situational. It is acquired over time from many sources, potent among these is the role model. Many nurses will admit to having been impressed with the skilled performance of a theatre nurse while handing instruments to a surgeon. The desire to emulate this can be a powerful motivator to learn. Quite often a nurse, while handing instruments to a surgeon, will be expected to maintain a managerial role within the theatre, maybe covering a whole suite. Becoming this skilled in such a specialised area is a recognition of the unique role of the theatre nurse. Castledine (1995) declares that, 'nurses in hospitals will create their own particular specialist domain' and this is a particularly important point for theatre nurses, who have seen their roles shared out to other disciplines. Observing theatre nurses carrying out their role successfully may be one way of attracting students towards making their career in theatres when they qualify.

Students are exposed to a number of specialist areas during their pre-registration preparation. It would seem a natural part of a surgical nursing experience to include a spell in theatre, indeed this always used to be part of nurse training. Experience of caring for patients in the operating theatre is no longer automatically included in nurse training programmes.

The current trend towards student centred learning and the exercise of student choice means that both student and teacher may concentrate more on the process of learning than its product (Shailer, 1997). Allowing students to choose elective clinical experiences emphasises the adult learning approach of the university system, and is welcomed by students (Grant, 1987; Shailer, 1997). The current trend towards reflection on experiences is also an attractive learning tool, which is very personal to the student (Richardson and Maltby, 1995) and should therefore be effective. For pre-registration students specialisation is not a pressing issue, but for currently qualified and practising nurses, continuing education programmes are their route to continued professional development. According to MacGregor and Dewar (1997) the current framework of post basic education:

> *should be a flexible vehicle by which individuals can gain expanded knowledge in a particular field of practice or can change professional direction if they wish.*

Post basic education is not restricted to prescribed nursing courses. A variety of educational opportunities are available through various routes and institutions.

Critical incidents and reflective practice

Operating theatres offer the student the opportunity to concentrate on the care of a single patient, while that patient is in the department. Being guided through a structured reflection of such an experience, by an experienced theatre nurse, has the potential to make a positive impression of specialist practice on student nurses (Smith, 1995) and retain a humanising influence in an area of high technology (Pearson, 1993). Personal development through the use of a reflective journal is a well established part of pre-registration nurse education (Richardson and Maltby, 1995). A possible danger in promoting reflective practice is that nurses may understandably conceal or be reluctant to discuss errors in practice. Meurier *et al* (1997) conducted a study which examined the causes and consequences of errors. They found a number of predisposing factors but were able to identify coping strategies which, within a supportive environment, 'were found to lead to positive changes in practice'. Reflection could usefully be a part of this process.

Developing specialists

Brown (1995) identifies a political agenda in the development of specialised and advanced nursing practitioners, asserting that it could be, 'an expediency measure aimed at conserving the expensive energies of doctors for more worthy work'. This argument can certainly be applied to the development of surgeon's assistant roles, but these roles have been welcomed and taken up by nurses, ODAs and ODPs. The roles are now recognised and courses supporting them are validated by the National Boards responsible for overseeing nurse education. Nurses may see such roles as a legitimate career opportunity, where their established knowledge of surgery can be put to good use. Surgeon's assistants do not need to be restricted to assisting in the operating theatre, but can be used to deliver truly holistic care for patients from referral to follow up and discharge (Williams, 1996b).

The Operating Room Nurses' Association of Canada (ORNAC) (1996) reports on the development of curricula for the roles of 'perioperative nurse anaesthesia' and 'perioperative nurse surgery', with the goal of:

> *The preparation of a practitioner who bases practice on advanced knowledge of nursing art and science, and on the content relevant to specialised health care from other disciplines.*

This is a world away from the subservient and doctor dominated vision of theatre nurses, where nurses will be encouraged to become:

> *reflective critical thinkers, self-directed lifelong learners and collaborative practitioners who function independently and interdependently within a multidisciplinary team.*

Sounds like theatre nursing utopia. Unfortunately, as will be shown in *Chapter 3*, it is not what some surgeons and anaesthetists want from theatre nurses.

An indication of how diverse and specialised operating theatre nursing has become can be seen in the *American Operating Room Nurses* (AORN) *Journal,* reporting on the Association's annual congress (*AORN Journal*, 1997). Nineteen networking groups met to discuss their individual specialised needs. These groups were not just collections of nurses from different surgical specialities, the groups included pre-admission planners, research, quality assessment, ethics and computers and information systems. This shows that American operating room nurses are dedicated to being in control of their working lives. They are clearly aware of the contribution nurses make to operating room care, and have their priorities on every agenda. United Kingdom theatre nurses have similar opportunities provided by NATN.

For operating theatre nurses to have a legitimate and continuing role, some sort of recognised career pathway would be helpful. This would involve not only further developing specialist knowledge and expertise, but also having current knowledge and skills acknowledged. This means 'tapping into the creative potential of staff' (Langstaff and Gray, 1997) and recognising the value of intuitive knowledge. The need for clear career pathways, and information on them is established by a long term research study (Robinson *et al*, 1997) which found uncertainty about career pathways was an important issue for nurses.

Conclusion

Nurse education up to registration provides a competent practitioner able to work autonomously in a variety of nursing situations. The nurse who decides to pursue a career in perioperative nursing will need to expand these basic competencies, and develop a further specialised knowledge base. The nursing basis of perioperative care also allows for a different kind of autonomous practice with patients who are vulnerable and undergoing what is probably one of the most significant experiences of their lives. This is a recognised and rewarding career pathway.

References

Brown R (1995) The politics of specialist/advanced practice: conflict or confusion? *Br J Nurs* **4**(16): 944–948

Castledine G (1995) Specialisation in nursing comes of age. *Br J Nurs* **4**(5): 295

Castledine G (1997) Framework for a clinical career structure in nursing. *Br J Nurs* **6**(5): 264–271

Conway J (1995) *Expert Nursing Knowledge as an Evolutionary Process*. Unpublished PhD thesis, University of Warwick, Coventry

Delamothe T (1988) Nursing grievances IV: Not a profession, not a career. *Br Med J* **296**, 23rd January: 271–274

Erikson G (1996) When the nurse holds the scalpel. *Br J Theatre Nurs* **6**(5): 48

Glen S (1995) Towards a new model of nursing education. *Nurse Ed Today* **15**: 90–95

Grant P (1987) An elective experience. *Nurs Times* **83**(33): 59–61

Hart G, Rotem A (1995) The clinical learning environment: Nurses' perceptions of professional development in clinical settings. *Nurse Ed Today* **15**(3): 3–9

Kolb D (1984) *Experiential Learning: Experience as the source of learning and developmen*t. Prentice Hall, New Jersey

Langstaff D, Gray B (1997) Flexible roles: a new model in nursing practice. *Br J Nurs* **6**(11): 635–638

Lawson N (1996) Irrelevant academic qualifications are an insult to nurses — and dangerous to their patients. *The Times*, 26th December

MacGregor J, Dewar K (1997) Opening up the options: making the inflexible into a flexible framework. *Nurse Ed Today* **17**(5): 502–507

Meurier C, Vincent C, Parmar D (1997) Learning from errors in nursing practice. *J Adv Nurs* **26**: 111–119

Neubaur J (1995) The value of nursing. *J Nurs Management* **3**: 301–305

Operating Room Nurses Association of Canada (1996) Blueprint for: Curricula Development for the Role of Perioperative Nurse Anaesthesia (PNA) and Perioperative Nurse Surgery (PNS). *Can Operating Room Nurses J* November/December: 16–20

Pearson A (1993) Guest editorial: Nursing, technology and the human condition. *J Adv Nurs* **18**: 165–167

Richardson G, Maynard A (1995) *Fewer Doctors? More Nurses? A review of the knowledge base of Doctor-Nurse Substitution.* University of York Centre for Health Economics, Discussion Paper 135

Richardson G, Maltby H (1995) Reflection-on-practice: enhancing student learning. *J Adv Nurs* **22**: 235–242

Robinson S, Murrells T, Marsland L (1997) Constructing clinical pathways in nursing: some issues for research and policy. *J Adv Nurs* **25**: 602–614,

Rogers C (1983) *Freedom to Learn for the 80s.* Merrill, Columbus, Ohio

Shailer B (1997) Clinical electives: the challenges and benefits of student choice. *Br J Nurs* **6**(10): 575–583

Smith C (1995) Evaluating nursing care: reflection on practice. *Prof Nurse* **10**(11): 723–724

Steinaker N, Bell M (1979) *The experiential taxonomy: A new approach to teaching and learning.* Academic Press, New York

Williams M (1996a) *Managing Continuing Education. A Consumers and Providers Point of View*. Quay Books, Mark Allen Publishing Limited, Dinton, Salisbury, Wiltshire

Williams M (1996b) The expanding role of the nurse in laparoscopic surgery. *Br J Theatre Nurs* **6**(4): 34–35

3
Great expectations

Chitwood and Swain (1992) define perioperative nursing as:

Providing care for the patient during a period of enforced dependency.

This is certainly true. Patients before, during and immediately after surgery and anaesthesia are highly dependent on a caring presence to protect them from harm. Nurses also have an advocacy role, to speak and act on behalf of the patient in order not only to protect them from physical harm but to protect their wider interests as well. These responsibilities are clearly set out in the UKCC's *Code of Conduct.* For nurses to carry out these responsibilities in operating theatres requires an understanding and appreciation of the roles and responsibilities of the other members of the theatre team.

The teamwork essential for operating theatre work raises expectations of nurses from surgeons and anaesthetists. Much debate has ensued over many years about what nurses in theatre actually do or should do, and whether in fact any nursing takes place there (Holmes, 1994). The author's research and experience leads to the belief that surgeons and anaesthetists expect nurses to facilitate the process of surgery, mainly by providing a continuous supply of patients at suitable intervals so that delay is minimised or eliminated. Further to this, it is expected that nurses will manage and incorporate changes to scheduled work, and generally establish a co-operative relationship between all disciplines (MacRae, 1995). With these thoughts in mind, the author interviewed surgeons and anaesthetists to find out what they expected from theatre nurses.

One surgeon, when asked what his expectations of nurses were, began by reviewing his experiences of what nurses did in wards. He observed that he did not greatly value the taking of 'a history', as he called it by nurses, although he conceded that many things of great importance to the patient could usefully be recorded by nurses, but felt that patients 'worries about the dog' had no place in 'the notes' (assumed to be the medical, not nursing, notes). In fact, this surgeon declared that he did not value the nursing process at all. This is an interesting point which highlights the differences between medicine and nursing, doctors are trained to diagnose and treat signs, symptoms and disease processes, nurses are trained to care holistically for patients.

The same surgeon did value 'nurses getting to know patients' so at least tentatively acknowledging the value of holistic care. This goes some way towards a reconciliation of roles, though the potential for conflict is evident. Continuity of care by the same nurses was highlighted as important by this surgeon, who believed that moving patients between areas (admission ward, surgical ward, high dependency) was confusing and frightening for patients, and should not be done without good reason. This surgeon stated that, 'when a patient is admitted to hospital, the first nurse you encounter is like a friend, but unfortunately you may not see the same nurse again due to shift patterns, days off and leave'. Here lies this surgeon's expectations of ward nurses, that they should be there all the time, comforting and caring while the doctor's interventions are being planned and delivered.

That's fine in a ward setting, but what expectations does he have of nurses in theatre? His opening remarks to this question revealed some surprises. Care was not high on this surgeon's agenda as the primary role for theatre nurses. He felt that the management role — sending for patients, organising equipment, making sure instrument sets were ready — was vital in ensuring that 'my time is not wasted'. This initially seemed like a pompous and arrogant remark but, on further reflection, some sense behind it becomes apparent. Operating theatre time is very expensive, efficiency in terms of cost as well as everything else is vital in the Health Service today. The author does not believe that this surgeon felt that only his time was important, but that everyone else's was too.

When asked if nurses were essential to operating theatres, and could their role be assumed by another discipline, a surgeon replied that he was sure he would miss them, without specifying why. Then followed a surprising revelation that in his opinion, men (whether they should be nurses or not he didn't say) would be more appropriate in theatre 'because they are so much more practical than women'. Women, he stated, 'get confused by the simplest things, men have a cultural background of being able to handle screws, levers and ratchets'. Women's attitudes to instruments he described as 'deplorable' in his experience, and felt that if he asked a man to 'get this fixed' then it would automatically get done. Men, apparently, have 'a practical attitude towards tools and, after all, surgery is the manipulation of tools... and it's the tools that do the job'. No mention was made of male nurses. This is a rather sad and stereotyped assumption from a very experienced surgeon for whom the author has a great deal of respect. It illustrates vividly the fact that operating theatre nurses and nursing are not always greatly valued or recognised for their knowledge and skills.

An anaesthetist when asked for his expectations of theatre nurses said that he expected them 'to run theatres'. When invited to expand on this he went on to describe a managerial and educational role for theatre nurses, and a caring role which he indicated should be directed towards surgeons and anaesthetists! Additionally, he expected the theatre nurse to promote good working relationships between staff, and generally assume an organisational role. Described in these terms, such a person need not necessarily be a nurse, and when this was pointed out, the anaesthetist said that he would not be happy for theatres to be managed by people other than nurses or ODPs. His rationale for this view was that the person in charge must have first hand knowledge and experience of theatre practices, and that it was not a job that just anyone could do.

The surgeons and anaesthetists quoted above appear to be demonstrating what Conway (1996) identifies as 'a form of oppression by medical staff in relation to nurses', expecting them to be compliant, flexible and obedient. There is clear evidence that gender stereotyping and 'a type of benign paternalism' (Conway, 1996) are the overriding criteria. The author's own experiences support this view.

Conclusion

It is tempting to resort to fighting talk, to become angry and disillusioned at such chauvinistic and pompous remarks. These are hopefully minority views, though personal experience and current observations lead to the conclusion that they are probably quite widespread. Fighting with the surgeons and anaesthetists will do nursing no good. Becoming well educated might be one answer. Knowledge is power. The medical profession is powerful because it has a well established and proven knowledge base. It also has much tighter control of entry to training and standards of practice than nursing. It is also led and dominated by men.

There are many surgeons and anaesthetists who regard nurses as their dependable, skilful and equal colleagues. We must encourage these people and seek to raise the consciousness of others. Women can be just as powerful and are possibly more subtle in their exercise of such power.

References

Chitwood L, Swain D (1992) *Perioperative Nursing. A Study and Revision Tool.* Springhouse Notes, Springhouse Corporation, Pennslyvannia

Conway J (1996) *Nursing Expertise and Advanced Practice.* Quay Books, Mark Allen Publishing Limited, Dinton, Salisbury, Wiltshire

Holmes L (1994) Theatre nursing (Part 1). *Br J Theatre Nurs* **4**(5): 11–15

MacRae W (1995) Anaesthesia and recovery. *Br J Theatre Nurs* **4**(12): 5

United Kingdom Central Council for Nursing, Midwifery and Health Visiting (1992) *Code of Professional Conduct*. UKCC, London

4

Preparing the perioperative workforce

We're all in this together...

Nurses have never had an exclusive claim to ownership of activities defined as 'nursing'. All over the world, sick and disabled people are 'nursed' by families, friends, religious orders and a multitude of others. There is no universally accepted definition of 'nursing', although attempts to develop one have been made. Caring, nurturing, supporting, feeding, and other activities form the mainstay of what is generally accepted as 'nursing care' — whoever is doing it. The United Kingdom has formalised nursing into a recognised role and supported this with training and education programmes leading to nursing qualifications. The present form of nurse training takes place in university schools of nursing, and leads to both a nursing and academic qualification on successful completion. This arrangement sends the message that nursing is a skilled undertaking requiring a significant knowledge base to support it. The duties carried out by non-nurses in support of nursing have been recognised with a range of National Vocational Qualifications (NVQs) in England and Wales and Scottish Vocational Qualifications (SVQs) in Scotland. The title usually given to these support workers is health care assistant (HCA).

Background to NVQs

Changes in the NHS, nurse education and a review of training standards were all taking place at the same time, between 1986 and 1988. Certainly politics was a major driving force in these changes, not only nationally but also within the European Community (Day, 1995).

In discussing the development and place of NVQs, Day (1995) points out that 'traditionally, professional and statutory bodies have had the responsibility for ensuring standards in education and training' but that NVQs were developed as a result of government policy. This begs the question of the potential political manipulation of nursing by government. Such a position does nothing to further nursing's cause to be recognised as a true profession. Because of the lack of clear boundaries to nursing care, much of what nurses have done as part of their role in the past has been included within the vocational training package. The government is anxious to promote training and qualifications for as much of the work-force as possible, and vocational qualifications have provided an ideal way to do this on a nationwide basis (Hevey, 1994). The focus of vocational training is skills, 'what candidates can do in real work settings' (Hevey, 1994). This contrasts sharply with the university academic base to nurse training, where hands on skills are supported by wide ranging theoretical and research-based knowledge. Some conflict of ideals is obvious — if nursing has handed over roles which apparently need skill but little knowledge, then is what is left 'real nursing'? What is the significance of what nurses did before they were supported by vocationally trained assistants? Hevey (1994) does not see this as a problem:

> *Some early forms of occupational standards at lower levels, however, encouraged a mechanistic 'check list' approach to assessment. There has also been much disinformation about deskilling, ignoring ethics and values and about losing any sense of the holistic nature of work roles and functions. All NVQs have had a bad press in the past.*

Examining the activities which nurses have traditionally carried out in nursing patients has led to some of these being delegated to non-nurses, on the basis that the skill and knowledge required to carry them out is less than that expected of a nurse. This also enables employers to save on labour costs: 'A major implication of the thrust to deliver less costly but high quality health care is the corresponding need to match skills to the task' (Pickersgill, 1998). Perioperative nurses should decide what are the boundaries of their practice, and what support staff can legitimately do, but in most operating suites these decisions reflect the organisational culture and financial constraints, as well as the preferences of surgeons and anaesthetists. This may be tellingly revealed in the constituents of appointment boards. Surgeons and anaesthetists are often involved in selecting applicants for nursing and operating department practitioner (ODP) posts, but not usually involved in appointing nurses and HCAs to positions outside theatres. Such situations may speak volumes about whose agenda is being followed.

At the same time, nursing is striving to change its image from one of self-sacrificing subservience to medicine to one of professional, researched and autonomous practice, providing holistic and individual patient care. Dividing nursing work into skilled and non-skilled activities is at odds with this holistic and individualised concept, though not everyone agrees with this. Rowden (1992) sees some nursing tasks as interchangeable between nurses and non-nurses, though he does concede that the practice of healthcare assistants needs to be supervised by qualified nurses. An emphasis on the tasks of nursing is a further erosion of professional status, leading to fragmented and ritualistic practice. Elliot (1994) sees potential for much conflict in this:

> *The profession has spent endless time justifying its position, arguing about models of care and how to document them, and forging links with higher education. But others were introducing systems to ensure that support staff will be 'qualified' to do actual tasks which were the foundations of our very profession in the first place.*

This situation is probably more clearly seen in operating theatres than anywhere else. Nurses have only themselves to blame for abdicating compartments of care which perhaps do not seem much like 'real' nursing, the best example being anaesthetic care. Having allowed others to take control, the situation is now probably beyond redemption.

In operating theatres it is often difficult to see any activities which would be readily recognised as 'nursing'. Anaesthesia, surgery and recovery are complex and intensive undertakings requiring very specialised skills, often carried out by two people working in partnership. For instance, the induction of anaesthesia requires that the anaesthetist has a skilled assistant, and the same is true of surgery. Because of the specialist nature of both anaesthesia and surgery, each has developed its own skilled helper role. This has led to a demarcation of roles which in some theatres acts to the detriment of continuous patient care. The skilled helper has become a significant contributor to the workforce but in some cases only within strictly confined areas. An overemphasis on skills development alone is all too easy in a highly technical and practical setting. To deny the cognitive and affective development of staff is to deny their individual and particular learning needs. While not exactly 'giving a monkey a gun', the current situation produces many potential areas for conflicts of interest and opposing philosophical views.

Perhaps in an attempt to mollify professional opinion, an amalgamation of vocational and professional education has been suggested. Storey *et al* (1995) reveal the possibility of incorporating NVQ Level 3 management into nurse pre-registration training as part of the branch programme. They conclude that, 'it is important that NVQs are not used as determining factors for successful completion of the diploma programme. They are used solely in contributing disciplines where there is a clear requirement for vocational competence at a level **below** that which could be expected of the nursing skills of diplomates'. A further interesting point regarding competence levels and NVQs is that Level 3 is accepted as an entry gate to nurse training, but qualified operating department practitioners (ODPs) at Level 3 can compete with qualified nurses for posts in operating theatres.

The varying levels of vocational qualifications and their performance based assessments may give rise to concerns about reliability, validity and potential threat to nurses as observed by Elliot (1994):

The whole NVQ package can be offered, monitored and assessed by non nurses. At Level 2 this may be appropriate. Level 3 however, contains well-identified nursing procedures. If allowed to proceed, managers with the inevitable calculators in hand will work out that one registered nurse will be sufficient in a care setting, ie. a group of wards, a nursing home, a community district... The role of the registered nurse will be to 'carry the can' when things go wrong and be the person liable in the eyes of the law.

This is probably being a little over dramatic, but the basic premise of the scope of accountability which nurses carry as a result of their registration cannot be ignored. Would you wish to be the only qualified nurse in an operating department staffed by NVQ qualified people? Registration for ODPs has long been debated and even promised, but seems no nearer. For the moment, ODPs are accountable for their actions in law and to their employer as we all are. They do not have to account for their practice to any other body, and therefore cannot be prevented from practising or have their qualification removed. Continuing education for ODPs is not a requirement, though most employers do encourage all theatre staff to expand their knowledge and keep practices up-to-date. The university system does not ignore vocational qualifications or learning gained from experience in practice. A mechanism of accreditation of prior learning (APL), accreditation of prior experiential learning (APEL), and accreditation of prior achievement (APA) enables people with vocational qualifications and experience in practice to have these recognised as part of academic awards. So the academic and vocational systems are not mutually exclusive and can compliment each other at all levels. There are some who foresee nursing as an all graduate profession in the future, and if this comes to pass, ODPs need not feel excluded or threatened as they too can access the academic pathway.

Warr *et al* (1998) researches the expansion of the nursing profession and anticipates an all graduate entry into practice for the future. They realise that this will require some other changes including 'delegation of professional nursing activities' but do not define these. There are also opportunities for nurses to expand their practice into semi-doctor roles (surgeon's assistant, nurse endoscopist). Warr *et al* see this as 'enabling people, at any time in their life, to gain access to the knowledge, skills and attitudes that are the basis of technical competence and self development'. Warr *et al* (1998) conclude:

> *The consummate reduction in numbers of highly skilled, professional nurses may force them into increasingly specialised roles. This could be the price nurses will have to pay for the increasing professionalisation of this once essentially vocational caring service.*

University preparation of nurses for registration is seen by some as 'clinically de-skilling' (Corbett, 1998) and leading to a displacement of nursing knowledge. This is completely at odds with the findings of Warr *et al*'s (1998) research study, but the article is not itself research-based. Corbett's (1998) extensive examination of the literature and a number of theoretical frameworks lead him to conclude:

> *Project 2000 has successfully 'uncoupled' two sets of needs, those of service and education, seen as necessary for enhancing educational standards and for the professionalisation of nursing.*
>
> Walby *et al*, 1994

Pickersgill (1998) supports Corbett's (1998) assertion that current nurse education is unsatisfactory, but takes the view that:

> *Graduate education is the norm in most western European countries and in Australia and the US. The standardisation of nurse education at degree level has enabled nurses to influence health legislation at both national and state level. Evidence from the medical profession suggests that a standardised and learned education is a potent unifying force.*

The author does not believe that nurses have to give up on delivering direct care to demonstrate specialised professional practice. There does not have to be a choice between knowing and doing, nursing needs both.

Conclusion

These similar criticisms but opposing solutions seem to leave nursing at a crossroads. Graduates, diplomats and vocational carers all seem to have the potential to assume the title 'nurse'. Nurses themselves must decide where their future lies, and elect the leaders who will take them there. There will never be a shortage of patients needing care, and increasingly those patients are being encouraged to demand higher standards of care. Both vocational and academic routes to qualification are available and will continue to develop. They are compatible and useful ways of obtaining both specialist and general qualifications. There is certainly enough evidence to suggest that a well qualified workforce provides better care than a non-qualified workforce (UKCC, 1994; Orme, 1992).

References

Corbett K (1998) The captive market in nurse education and the displacement of nursing knowledge. *J Adv Nurs* **28**(3): 524–531

Day M (1995) Vocational training: its role in nursing. *Nurs Standard* **9**(51): 34–37

Elliot M (1994) NVQ for the dole? *Nurs Standard* **8**(48): 36

Hevey D (1994) NVQs at the leading edge. *Nurs Standard* **8**(31): 20–22

Orme L (1992) Project paper six. *Continuing professional education in the context of health care*. A report for the English National Board for Nursing, Midwifery and Health Visiting, ENB, London,

Pickersgill F (1998) Time to catch up. *Nurs Standard* **12**(37): 26–27

Rowden R (1992) More input required. *Nurs Times* **88**(33): 27–28

Storey L, Greenham S, Martin E (1995) NVQs as part of the pre-registration diploma. *Nurs Times*: 34–35

United Kingdom Central Council for Nursing, Midwifery and
Health Visiting (1994) *The Future of Professional Practice —
the Council's standards for Education and Practice following
Registration. Position Statement on Policy and
Implementation.* UKCC, London

Walby S, Greenwell J, Mackay L, Soothill K (1994) *Medicine and
Nursing. Professions in a changing health service.* Sage
Publications, London

Warr J, Gobbi M, Johnson S (1998) Expanding the nursing
profession. *Nurs Standard* **12**(31): 44–47

5

Managing perioperative care

Patients as consumers of healthcare

The internal market in healthcare introduced by the Conservative government in 1990 instigated the purchase and provision of health services. Buying and selling health services took place between providers — that was any public or private organisation, Trust, or health authority who delivered healthcare services — and purchasers, who could be any public or private organisation, Trust or health authority who needed to supply healthcare services to patients. Thus, either party involved in the transaction could be a purchaser, provider or both, depending on who needed which services. This situation was supposed to promote quality and choice for consumers by influencing providers to be efficient so that they would attract more consumers. In fact, patients had little or no voice in this process because choices were made for them by GPs who, if they were fundholders, would usually opt for the cheapest provider.

The current Government is pledged to dismantle this market and eliminate competition between providers. In the United States, where healthcare is largely insurance based, then the marketing of health services has an overt commercial appearance, and the customer is king (Gregory Dawes, 1998). The UK National Health Service is probably the most significant element in our welfare state, and the one we are most likely to use. It swallows up huge amounts of our money and in using the service people have the right to expect good value for their pre-paid money. Therefore, the conception of patients as consumers of healthcare is an appropriate one.

Surgery is probably the most easily 'packaged' type of health service and as such lends itself to becoming a saleable commodity. The danger is that operating theatres and the staff within them could become the shelf stackers and checkout clerks of a kind of surgical supermarket, with the patients simply wheeled through in those ubiquitous wire trolleys. Nurses would do well to remember that it is people who have operations, and every person is unique. Nurses have a responsibility to act as the patient's advocate during surgery, a responsibility that cannot be ignored in the name of 'productivity'.

Influences on nursing practice

Observing theatre nurses going about their work might lead to the conclusion that they provide a service for surgeons and anaesthetists as much as patients. This is what the surgeons and anaesthetists in the earlier chapter wanted, and it appears that nurses are playing into their hands. To redress the balance, an examination of some of the theoretical influences on nursing practice is appropriate.

Nursing lays claim to a number of theoretically based models on which to base care, such models providing a framework within which care is delivered. Alongside these models, there is also the 'nursing process' — a systematic, problem solving approach to individualised patient care. Farmer (1986) describes nursing care as being:

> *...based on a critical analysis of patients' requirements for effective living, and their ability or otherwise to meet these requirements independently, rather than on speculation or assumption.*

This would seem to be a rational approach, presenting no difficulties as the basis of caring for patients in theatre. As for the nursing process, the stages of assessment, planning, delivering and evaluating care are different in an operating theatre context because of the nurses' limited access to the patient prior to surgery. Accepting that 'the nursing process is the underlying scheme that provides direction to nursing care. It is the essence of professional practice' (Stanton *et al*, 1990), then theatre nurses need to clearly establish and record how and when they assess, plan, deliver and evaluate patient care, and demonstrate a sound basis for that care. These themes will be discussed later, following an examination of some of the theoretical, psychological and social influences on nursing practice.

Nursing models

A recognised nursing model may be one basis for practice, although there is a temptation to use the model outline as the format for assessment (eg. activities of living) and not carry through the operationalisation of the other elements of the model. There is also the temptation to take up the model used by the rest of the hospital, whether or not it fits the requirements for perioperative care. These theoretical arguments may seem academic and unnecessary, where patients are undergoing possibly the most significant experience of their entire lives. Such observations may lead to theatre nurses rejecting models in favour of an approach which is centred on meeting human needs.

Meeting human needs

Maslow's hierarchy of basic human needs (Potter and Perry, 1995) could be used as the foundation for meeting the individual needs of patients with a variety of levels of dependence, and over a wide age range. The hierarchy provides a generalised view of needs priorities, and in using it as the basis for perioperative nursing, priorities may be established, fulfilled and re-established as dependency changes (Potter and Perry, 1995). In using any sort of model or framework for care, perioperative nurses are declaring ownership of that care and separating it from the diagnostic and therapeutic imperatives of the medical model. The need to do this may be related to the complexity of the relationships between doctors and nurses and the game playing referred to in *Chapter 1.*

The medical model

Trying to break free of the 'servant and master' relationship will occupy nurses for many generations to come, as the revelations in *Chapter 3* show. Such subservient and task oriented cultures do nurses and nursing no favours or, indeed, patients (Tanner, 1998). Further support for nursing autonomy comes from Jolley and Brycznska (1993):

> *The handmaiden mentality and tasks of nurses are not natural female responses to human needs. They are the outcome of a system which openly supports separation between cure and care, while covertly relying on nurses to fill the gap in between.*

The medical profession, in operating theatres or anywhere else, are not going to change their position on this. Though there are many doctors who willingly and openly acknowledge the role nursing plays in patient outcomes, many do not. The lack of solid, scientific credibility for nursing in terms of measured outcomes is one reason for this. Nursing research is in its infancy, and much of the available research is qualitative. Presenting this to the medical profession whose practice is predominantly based on quantitative, controlled trials does little to further nursing's cause. A dismissal of nursing research as 'emotional claptrap' has been the author's experience of trying to explain qualitative enquiry to a doctor. Coupled with the gender prejudices discussed earlier, there are no easy answers here, but giving up is not the answer either. Theatre nurses need to examine their own practice from a variety of perspectives, record it accurately and declare ownership of it.

Varona (1997) offers a fascinating and unique examination of the ways in which theatre nurses approach their patients, dividing them into 'technical nurses' and 'caring nurses' by using sample dialogues with patients. Such insights need to be considered by theatre nurses because they put individual patient care into sharp focus.

An interesting and research based view on the use of nursing models for theatre nursing is offered by Tanner (1998) who advises:

> *Before implementing any nursing model in theatre, theatre nurses should examine their own beliefs, values and attitudes and devise a model that complements their needs.*

Evidence-based practice

Research into nursing is the way evidence for practice is generated. Research and its application has to be the most effective long term strategy for establishing the credibility of nursing practice. There is resistance within the profession to be overcome before this can be realised as many nurses still do not attach importance to research findings, and some actively resist their application (Chapman, 1996). Even for the most committed nurse, finding, understanding and applying research to practice may be a long, hard and frustrating task. Establishing a basis for practice founded on a nursing model or a psychological one such as Maslow, and supporting practice with research, has to be followed by a systematic, problem focused process which begins with assessment of each patient's problems. The process of research and its translation into practice is explored more fully in *Chapter 5*.

Opportunities for assessment

In order for theatre nurses to make their assessment of patients' actual and potential problems for the duration of their stay in theatre they need to find opportunities to meet the patient and gather the necessary information. This can be the first stumbling block. Due to the pressure to treat as many patients as possible and to make maximum use of the available beds, most patients are now admitted on the morning of the day on which their surgery is to take place. A pre-operative visit from the theatre nurse is difficult to arrange in such circumstances, though some determined and committed units do manage it.

What can be achieved during a short visit to the patient before they come to theatre is limited but can be significant if the will to carry it out is there (Wicker, 1995). In any case, in order to nurse the patient safely and effectively during their stay in the theatre suite, assessment of the patient has to take place on first meeting and at intervals afterwards. Pre-assessment clinics for day surgery (Neasham, 1996) and in-patient surgery offer the opportunity for theatre nurses to meet patients prior to surgery and begin the assessment process.

Assessment is not a once and for all event. An initial assessment describes the current situation, which will inevitably change with the administration of anaesthesia, the transfer to theatre, surgery and recovery. Nevertheless, the first assessment is important as it must provide the basis for planning to meet the patient's needs. Each member of the caring team will make an assessment of the patient as care is transferred. Few of these assessments will be recorded. This lack of solid evidence is one reason why operating theatre nursing is deemed to be 'invisible' or not really nursing at all. Operating room nurses in the United States have realised that in order to demonstrate ownership of perioperative care they must clearly identify what they do and communicate this to other nurses and colleagues (Morton, 1998).

Much criticism of the nursing process stems from a misconception that the paperwork takes precedence over delivering care. No sensible nurse would put filling in forms before patient care and safety. Assessment in emergency situations recognises and prioritises immediate needs, delivers interventions which stabilise the situation and reassesses the new situation. Plans for care based on a comprehensive and prioritised assessment should offer the patient a safe pathway through the operating department.

Planning patient care

Based on information from assessment, achievable goals for patient care are set. In most nursing situations the goals will be met by the patient, but in operating theatres, goals may be set which the nurses have to meet. For example, the conscious and mobile patient with intact skin and a low risk of pressure damage will be at a greatly increased risk when immobilised by anaesthesia and positioned on an operating table for several hours. Therefore a plan of care which recognises the increased risk will require the nurse to deliver suitable interventions to prevent skin damage. Recognising actual and potential nursing problems which patients may have in operating theatres is the very essence of theatre nursing. These problems are the ones nursing interventions are required to deal with. They may or may not be directly related to the surgery and anaesthesia. American nurses refer to such problems as 'nursing diagnoses', defining this term as:

> *The identification of the human responses and resource limitations of the client for the general purpose of identifying and directing nursing care.*
>
> Stanton *et al*, 1990

Though rather wordy this does fit in with the more usual UK definition of 'patient problems'. Identifying problems and ways to solve them is the basis of planning nursing care. Planning patient care has recently assumed a greater significance with the development of clinical pathways (Fujihara-Isozaki and Fahndrick, 1998).

Becoming involved in multidisciplinary activities such as planning clinical pathways is another means by which theatre nurses may stake their claim to ownership of perioperative care. The emergence of clinical governance will bring into sharp focus the contributions of all staff to patient outcomes. Effective clinical pathways for surgical patients may provide the key to streamlining services, containing costs and promoting efficiency (Fujihara-Isozaki and Fahndrick, 1998). Theatre nurses must make their presence felt in designing clinical pathways, and ensure their involvement when patient care is recorded.

Implementing patient care

This means carrying out the plan of care produced from the assessment. In practice, a written plan with measurable goals is rare for operating theatre nurses, although some theatres use pre-printed core care plans which are individualised by the addition of patient specific information. The lack of a written plan does not mean that care is not delivered, indeed, operating theatre nurses have the relative luxury of only being expected to look after one patient at a time and do so in co-operation with other disciplines. As discussed earlier, the philosophy and underpinning values of those delivering care and the institution in which care is delivered will influence the actions taken in delivering care (Stanton *et al*, 1990).

Taking the time to stand back and reflect on practice allows an appreciation of just what it is that theatre nurses do and why they do it. This can be a significant, illuminating and educational process. An observation that, 'traditionally nursing was subservient to other professions such as doctors. For many of us this has resulted in a legacy of non-assertiveness...' (Glaze, 1999) may lead operating theatre nurses to question exactly what it is they do in delivering care. When challenged to define or even relate what 'theatre nursing' consists of, it may be difficult to come up with convincing answers. Wicker (1997) describes the variety and overlap of roles within the operating department and concludes that the survival or not of nurses as a part of the team delivering patient care is in their own hands. Saying that nurses 'care' is not enough, though the context of caring in the operating theatre was eloquently defined and supported by West (1993).

In addition to reflecting on practice, operating theatre nurses need to be aware of what is recorded about patient care. Nursing records are subjected to audit, and Trusts who cannot see what their theatre nurses are doing from nursing records are unlikely to value or support those nurses. Theatre nurses should take every opportunity to reflect on their contribution to patient care, and on the visibility or otherwise of nursing actions. Patients undoubtedly receive care in operating theatres and, as nursing cannot claim an exclusive role in delivering this, the implementation and recording of nursing on care plans assumes a greater importance.

Evaluating patient care

This vital part of the care process is probably the most neglected. Having planned and delivered care, evaluation is essential to complete the process. Assuming that planned interventions have been delivered and that they worked is not good enough. Evaluation will demonstrate what has been effective and, more importantly, what has not.

Evaluation has much in common with assessment. The difference between assessment and evaluation is assessment begins with no prior knowledge of the patient and their situation, whereas evaluation is based on the information gained at assessment compared to information collected after nursing interventions have been delivered. Marriner (1983) defines evaluation thus, 'evaluation of patient progress involves evaluation of goal achievement and reassessment of the care plan'.

Like assessment, evaluation has its priorities. The nurse evaluating the skin condition of a patient on transfer from the operating table to bed or trolley will want to know how the previously intact skin has reacted to hours of sustained dependence in one position — did the pressure relieving aids work? Is the skin red, pale, bruised? marked by covers or sheets? Is some further action necessary? These questions are all part of the evaluation process and need to be applied to every goal identified in the care plan.

Conclusion

Perioperative nursing care needs to be based on something, otherwise it becomes a collection of isolated tasks which could be delegated to a number of different people, qualified and unqualified, and may or may not meet patients' needs. Whatever care is based on, comprehensively recording the giving of that care serves not only to inform the next person who attends the patient, but also reflects the skill, knowledge and attitudes of those who have delivered it. Records of care are a means of evaluating quality, as well as providing audit data for a number of different reasons. They are also a professional record that care has been delivered.

If the only demonstrable evidence of perioperative nursing actually existing is the theatre care plan, then this document assumes an even greater professional importance. If you feel that your current theatre nursing documents do not reflect the care you deliver as well as they might, then the imperative to reform them and make your nursing visible is yours. The advent of clinical governance and the relentless audit process which informs it are a timely impetus for perioperative nurses to demonstrate what they contribute to patient outcomes.

References

Chapman H (1996) Why do nurses not make use of a solid research base? *Nurs Times* **92**(3): 38–39

Farmer E (1986) Exploring the Issues. In: Kershaw B, Salvage J (eds) *Models for Nursing*. John Wiley & Sons, Chichester

Fujihara-Isozaki L, Fahndrick J (1998) Clinical pathways — a perioperative application *AORN Journal* **67**(2): 376–392

Glaze J (1999) The reflective practitioner part 5: Reflecting on interpersonal and professional knowledge. *Br J Theatre Nurs* **9**(2): 64–69

Gregory Dawes B (1998) What every perioperative nurse should know about customers. *AORN Journal* **67**(5): 932–935

Jolley M, Brykcznska G (eds) (1993) *Nursing: Its hidden agendas*. Edward Arnold, London

Marriner A (1983) *The Nursing Process. A Scientific Approach to Nursing Care*. 3rd edn. CV Mosby, London

Morton P (1998) Data elements are the key to defining perioperative activities. *AORN J* **68**(5): 861–862

Neasham J (1996) Nurse led pre-assessment clinics. *Br J Theatre Nurs* **6**(8): 5–10

Potter P, Perry A (1995) *Foundations in Nursing, Theory and Practice*, Hazel Heath (ed). Mosby, London

Stanton M, Paul C, Reeves J (1990) An Overview of the Nursing Process. In: George J (ed) *Nursing Theories; The Basis for Professional Practice*. 3rd edn. Prentice Hall, London: chap 2

Tanner J (1998) The appropriateness of nursing models for theatre nurses. *Br J Theatre Nurs* **8**(8): 17–20

Varona L (1997) The perioperative nurse — carer or technician? *Br J Theatre Nurs* **7**(8): 10–13

West B (1993) Caring — the essence of theatre nursing. *Br J Theatre Nurs* **3**(9): 16–22

Wicker P (1995) Pre-operative visiting — making it work. *Br J Theatre Nurs* **5**(7): 16–20

Wicker P (1997) Overlapping roles in the operating department. *Nurs Standard* **11**(20): 44–45

6

Minimal access surgery, day surgery and perioperative nursing roles

Taylor and Wellwood (1997) in describing the principles of laparoscopic or minimal access surgery say:

> *The surgeon seeks to replicate the 'open' operation whilst dispensing with a large wound and its attendant pain and morbidity.*

They go on to describe in some detail a number of procedures which are amenable to the technique, but end with the statement, 'all of these procedures must be shown to be at least as safe and effective as the conventional approach before any recommendations for their widespread adoption can be made'. It is this final remark that provokes the thought that minimal access surgery seems to have been taken up with unseemly haste due to its perceived benefits but perhaps without due consideration of its limitations. This chapter examines a number of views and evaluates the effects of them on perioperative nursing.

Minimal access surgery

The recent rapid expansion of minimal access surgery has led to increased demands on perioperative staff not only to treat more patients but to master new skills in electronic and video technology (Phillips, 1996), as well as mastering the intricacies of new, complex and expensive instrumentation. Minimal access surgery now encompasses treatments carried out via flexible endoscopes as well as those performed via rigid endoscopes. A wide variety of surgery, once requiring extensive open procedures and intensive care is now possible via minimal access techniques (Valdes and Boudreau, 1996; Woerth *et al*, 1997; Rogers and Cox, 1998).

Alongside this has come the development of clinical pathways and the implication that 'quality improvement can be achieved through reduction in process variations' (Fujihara-Isozaki *et al*, 1998). It is interesting to note that this rapid expansion and adoption of a surgical technique has taken place against an almost complete absence of evidence of its safety and effectiveness compared to traditional open surgery. One piece of research comparing open versus laparoscopic inguinal hernia repair found the open method to be cheaper but the laparoscopic technique resulted in less infection and was more acceptable to patients (Wellwood *et al*, 1998). There are other financial concerns for nurses regarding single use items and the propensity for pressure to reuse them (Phillips, 1996). The research done by Wilmer, McEnteggart and Rogers (1997) found that 27% of staff in their sample of 127 nurses responsible for minimal access surgery instruments would resterilise single use instruments on request. Even more disturbing was the revelation that one respondent in the private sector had deliberately destroyed single use instruments to prevent them being removed for use in the NHS. Questions of accountability, risk management and patient safety loom large in this debate. The temptation to make operating theatres and day surgery units into surgical production lines seems ever present.

Not everyone is happy with the rapid expansion of minimal access surgery. Kapoor (1997) puts this down to 'general surgeons were enamoured and the patients attracted by a new technique. To this was added an enormous commercial push given by instrument manufacturers and the unusual publicity in the mass media'. This seems to be implying that we were sold something that had not been fully evaluated. While admitting the declared advantages of minimal access cholecystectomy Kapoor (1997) goes on to quote a randomised controlled trial which showed that laparoscopic cholecystectomy does not actually live up to these, and that the minimal access procedure takes longer, requires more specialised expensive instruments, and requires more expertise to perform. Johnson (1999) reflects on laparoscopic and minimally invasive surgery in even more alarming terms, citing Cusheri's (1995) condemnation, 'the biggest unaudited free-for-all in the history of surgery'. Perioperative nurses may feel that these debates do not directly concern them, but there is certainly a case for being aware of the wider implications of new surgical techniques which nurses and other taxpayers are funding.

Perioperative nursing roles

In spite of the problems highlighted above there is no doubt that reducing waiting times for surgery and in-patient admissions are welcomed by patients as well as managers and politicians. Minimal access surgery has played a major role in this. For perioperative nurses the development of minimal access surgery has offered:

> *...the opportunity to break the shackles of traditional roles in theatre and become actively involved in perioperative care. They can become independent, autonomous practitioners and make sure that a strong nursing presence remains in theatres to protect the needs of the patient.*

> Cabellero, 1998

These are the words of a nurse who has taken on a new role as a laparoscopic nurse practitioner. The role allows her to have a considerable degree of professional freedom in deciding on treatment options and helping to care for patients requiring cholecystectomy. Having witnessed this nurse in action (Williams, 1996), the author has nothing but admiration for the way she has developed the role and for the way in which perioperative nursing is enhanced within it, though not everyone agrees that this is a legitimate pathway for nursing to develop.

Concerns about the development of specialist nurse practitioner roles are raised by Castledine (1995) who suggests that nurses are perhaps too readily taking on roles formerly done by medical staff in order to relieve the pressure on junior doctors and to reduce costs. These are not exclusively British concerns (Hlozek *et al*, 1998). At the heart of the debate is the question of the quality of patient care and best use of limited resources. A training needs analysis carried out by Norfolk and Norwich Healthcare NHS Trust recommended that 'the trust's education strategy should be patient focused, driven by needs and measured by outcomes' (Edwards and Keeley, 1998). Edwards and Keeley (1998) admit that the reduction in junior doctors' hours was an influencing factor, and describe a number of developments offered to staff as a result. One of these was the opportunity to become a surgical assistant, which they define as 'recognised nationally as an interface between doctors and nurses in the operating theatre environment'. Nurses will choose whether or not to take up these roles for themselves. Arguments about being second class doctors or first class nurses are contextually related and will be decided by individuals. No-one has yet pointed a gun at a perioperative nurse and said, 'you will learn how to be a surgical assistant or else'. The current and chronic shortage of nurses and other staff in operating departments will ensure there is a continuing role for them in many capacities. Surgery will continue to develop new techniques which perioperative nurses will have to become familiar with in order to provide skilled help to surgeons and patients.

The development of new techniques brings up the question of learning how to become competent in them. For surgeons, Sackier (1997) advocates the traditional apprentice-ship method, 'from their senior colleagues by the same method one would learn open surgery'. This is right and proper for surgeons who have patients' lives and bodies in their hands. What of the nurse handling the instruments? The instrument manufacturers do provide courses, but these may not be accessible to all nurses. Being 'taken through' the new set just before you are expected to use it, by a colleague who had one or two days away from the workplace to learn all the ramifications is a poor substitute. The required learning extends beyond competent handling during surgery. Nurses may also be expected to dismantle, clean, sterilise, check and reassemble instruments.

All of this takes place against a background of professional accountability, waiting lists for surgery and pressure to keep patients out of hospital by increasing the number of operations done as day cases. Perioperative nurses are rising to this challenge by taking on a more holistic role in preparing and caring for patients before, during and after surgery. This is especially apparent in day surgery. A clear example of how successful such an approach can be is described by Quinn and Ludkin (1997) who are part of a team which has instituted a direct access hysteroscopy service in Bradford. They declare 'the hysteroscopy team is committed to a specific interest in women's health, and its philosophy is to give women informed choices to enable them to take charge of their own health'. There could be no better testimonial to the cause of perioperative nursing.

Day surgery

Being able to go home at the end of the day on which you had an operation may be a very attractive option for patients. The impetus for more and more patients to be treated this way is driven by 'both dubious and desirable' considerations (West and Lyon, 1995). Cost is undoubtedly one of these considerations and waiting lists another. Keeping people out of hospital and treating more of them are major considerations of the NHS today. Perioperative nurses are contributing to day surgery by becoming involved with patients at an earlier stage, and by being a continuous presence throughout the patient's stay. Beaumont (1997) describes an innovative project where nurses have taken on the assessment of patients for day case surgery. Following intensive and continuing education in this role, nurses now interview and examine patients and decide on their suitability or not for day case surgery. An audit of patient satisfaction involving 129 patients showed that patients were happy with the nurse led service. Audit data on patient satisfaction is now collected continuously and collated at six-monthly intervals. Though this single example is not sufficiently large to be generally applicable, the results are encouraging and lead Beaumont (1997) to declare, 'It is our intention to continue to review our service and maintain the innovative, high quality service we feel we now provide'.

Mason (1998) describes how the day surgery unit in Wolverhampton measures patient satisfaction with a telephone call to patients on the day following surgery. From this audit data perioperative nurses were able to highlight a problem with postoperative analgesia soon after the unit opened. Once identified, a cause of this problem became apparent and a change in analgesia prescribing was made. These examples show how nurses are able to contribute significantly to the quality of the patients' experience of day surgery, before and after the event.

Beaumont (1997) feels that there is room for more innovation for perioperative nurses in day surgery, expanding the assessment role into a full one-stop preoperative service including phlebotomy and ECG. Mason (1998) realistically suggests that as nurses are a finite resource, concentrating nursing efforts on improving patient satisfaction after discharge is both feasible and useful. West and Lyon (1995) point out:

> *If the responsibility for post-operative care should shift to the home care situation then it is suggested that surgical nurses fully explore the scope of professional practice and redirect their concerns to the support of the patient and carer before and after surgery.*

This is indeed the comprehensive holistic approach, and is probably a legitimate development of perioperative nursing. What is certain is that perioperative nurses, with proper education and support, are capable of contributing far more than they do at the moment to patient care.

Conclusion

Minimal access surgery has had major impact on surgery in the United Kingdom over the last ten years. It has been taken up, developed and expanded to the point where it is now an accepted surgical technique commonplace in most hospitals. Shorter patient stays and an increase in day surgery have been made possible. Minimal access surgery, and therapeutic procedures done via flexible endoscopes have transformed the treatment of some conditions which previously required extensive open procedures. No one would deny that this is a significant surgical advance.

Surgeons have had to develop new skills to operate via telescopes, and nurses have had to become expert camera operators as well as technicians. The instrumentation for minimal access surgery is complex and still developing. All of this presents challenges for perioperative nurses, not only to master the skills and knowledge involved, but to maintain a patient care focus where it is so easy to lose the patient in the technology.

References

Beaumont S (1997) Pre-operative assessment for day case surgery: a patient centred service. *Br J Theatre Nurs* 7(9): 9–13

Cabellero C (1998) The role of the laparoscopic nurse practitioner. *Nurs Standard* 12(44): 43–44

Castledine G (1995) Specialisation in nursing comes of age. *Br J Nurs* 4(5): 295

Cushieri A (1995) Whither minimal access surgery tribulations and expectations. *Am J Surg* 169: 9–19

Edwards C, Keeley O (1998) Competency-based learning for the surgical assistant. *Nurs Standard* 12(20): 44–47

Fujihara-Isozaki L, Fahndrick J (1998) Clinical pathways — a perioperative application *AORN Journal* 67(2): 376–392

Hlozek C, Zacharias W, Mizner K (1998) RN first assistants expand their perioperative role. *AORN Journal* 67(3): 560–566

Johnson A (1999) Laparoscopic surgery. *Br J Theatre Nurs* **9**(3): 119–123

Kapoor V (1997) 'Lap chole' — the other side of the coin. *Surgery* **15**: 192

Mason L (1998) Day surgery: improving care through follow up contact. *Br J Theatre Nurs* **8**(6): 11–13

Phillps K (1996) Issues of quality in minimal access surgery. *Nurs Standard* **11**(3): 52–53

Quinn P, Ludkin H (1997) Bradford's direct access hysteroscopy service. *Br J Theatre Nurs* **6**(10): 5–9

Rogers M, Cox J (1998) Laparoscopic paraoesophaegeal hernia repair with Nissen fundoplication. *AORN J* **67**(3): 536–551

Sackier J (1997) Protocols for training in minimally invasive surgery. *Surgery* **15**: 273–276

Taylor H, Wellwood J (1997) Principles and present status of laparoscopic general surgery. *Surgery* **15**: 73–75

Valdes M, Boudreau S (1996) Video-assisted thorascopic ligation of patent ductus arteriosus in children. *AORN J* **64**(4): 526–535

Wellwood J, Sculpher M, Stoker D *et al* (1998) Randomised controlled trial of laparoscopic versus open mesh repair for inguinal hernia: outcome and cost. *Br Med J* **317**(7151): 103–110

West B, Lyon M (1995) Day surgery: cheap option or challenge to care? *Br J Theatre Nurs* **5**(1): 5–8

Williams M (1996) The expanding role of the nurse in laparoscopic surgery. *Br J Theatre Nurs* **6**(4): 34–35

Wilmer S, McEnteggart K, Rogers J (1997) Reuse of single use items in minimal access surgery. *Br J Theatre Nurs* **7**(3): 11–13

Woerth S, Cranfil J, Neal J (1997) A collaborative approach to minimally invasive direct coronary artery bypass. *AORN J* **66**(6): 994–1001

7
Research not rituals

Basing practice on sound research is an important measure of nursing's credibility. Finding research specific to operating theatre nursing is not always easy. A search of the major sources of published nursing research in UK journals reveals a lack of material, research-based or other, related to perioperative nursing. The *British Journal of Theatre Nursing* published by NATN provides a voice for perioperative nurses as well as a platform for disseminating knowledge and research. More is always needed. Only perioperative nurses themselves can fill this gap.

Perhaps coinciding with this is the shortage of UK books on perioperative nursing. American publications are available, but the principles of practice put forward do not necessarily translate easily into the NHS system. Research from the United States may be applicable to UK healthcare settings, and there is certainly a lot more of it published. Perhaps the insurance driven base of healthcare in the United States promotes a more questioning approach. Questioning and challenging current practice requires the development of critical thinking skills which may be seen as 'common sense' or 'problem solving' (Dobrzykowski, 1994) but, this needs to be encouraged in order for perioperative nurses to deal with the increasing complexities of healthcare (Howenstein *et al*, 1996).

Being able to support practice with research is now seen as a measure of quality affecting the commissioning and contracting process (Dawson, 1995). The importance of a soundly based and multiprofessional audit is also seen as vital in forming the knowledge base for practice and ensuring quality (Kitson, 1996). Although audit differs from research in that it provides information on the current state of affairs rather than creating new knowledge or answering a specific question, audit data can form an important part of the research process.

Research is about asking questions and finding answers. Many nurses are put off by the language of research, or see it as complex and beyond their understanding. A better understanding of what research is and why nursing needs it may promote a readier acceptance to seek, read and apply it.

Why do we need research?

A global view of research and its place in society comes from Morse and Field (1996):

> *It is the means by which discoveries are made, ideas are confirmed or refuted, events controlled or predicted and theory developed or refined.*

If that seems rather academic and perhaps remote, then consider the more prosaic Polit and Hungler (1989) reasoning: 'research questions help nurses to provide more effective nursing care and to document the unique role that nursing plays in the healthcare system'. There are many more published sources which support the use of research for nursing practice (Watson, 1981; Chapman, 1996; Mead, 1996).

Most nurses now agree that the professional basis for practice has to be sustainable, reasoned and proven knowledge, but agreeing and doing are often far apart. Before research can be translated into practice some questions have to be answered. Nurses need to be sure of the extent to which any research results are applicable to practice situations. There is a danger in assuming that all research is applicable in the situations to which it is relevant, and that results can always be replicated. It is also worth noting that nursing research is still in its relative infancy, whereas medicine has research dating back to 1543 (Mead, 1996).

Not every nurse will have the inclination or opportunity to conduct research, this makes adopting and using the research of other nurses even more important. In order to adopt research-based practices, nurses must be able to read, understand and critique published research. Such understanding comes from a familiarity with the basic structure of the research process.

Ethics

Before any research can begin the researcher must ensure that the rights, freedoms and confidentiality of the research subjects are respected and protected. All participants in a research study must remain anonymous, and the data collected from them must be used only for the study and for no other purpose (Creswell, 1994). Ethical rules apply even if human subjects are not directly involved, for instance where data is retrieved from patient records. Collecting data from or about human subjects is an intrusion, however small, into their personal life and researchers must remember that it is being collected for the common good, not the subject's (Polit and Hungler, 1989). The ethical rules are applicable to all human subjects, whether they are members of staff or patients.

Hospitals and universities have ethical committees who examine all proposed research. Permission to carry out a study must be obtained from the appropriate ethical committee. This may entail research studies being redesigned in order to meet ethical requirements and protect participants. The informed consent of participants must be obtained, and they must also be aware of their right to withdraw from the study at any time.

Ethical committees may ask researchers to justify their proposals as well as their methods. A problem or issue which interests a research student may appear superficial and unimportant to an ethical committee. Research is about adding to the total sum of knowledge as well as seeking answers to questions and solutions to problems. Before proceeding to apply for ethical approval, research students must take all of this into account and be prepared to modify their proposal. Students undertaking research are usually supervised, and the supervisor will act as guide through this process as well as through the study.

Research questions

Research sets out to answer questions or solve problems. Medical research such as drug trials sets out to prove if one drug is more effective than another or a placebo. This type of research is seeking a definitive answer — whether the drug works or not. This is quantitative or scientific research, and it usually focuses on measurable or clear-cut parameters. Experiments, where one item is compared against another, or against a control group, are typical of quantitative research. Surveys which demonstrate how much, how often, or how many times something happens are also examples of quantitative research. There are many other examples of quantitative research methods described in research text-books. An example of a research question which could be answered by quantitative research would be: how much body heat do adult patients lose in the first hour of surgery under general anaesthetic? Polit and Hungler (1987) summarise quantitative research as:

> *The scientific approach to inquiry refers to a general set of orderly, disciplined procedures used to acquire dependable and useful information.*

In nursing, the questions and problems often do not lend themselves to such clear-cut and precise examination. Nursing questions are often about why things happen the way they do, or how attitudes are formed or affect the way things are done. Qualitative research is the way in which such questions are investigated. These questions often call for an exploration of a subject or problem in order to find a solution or to increase the knowledge about a subject. An appropriate description comes from Polit and Hungler (1989):

> *Qualitative research is often based on the premise that knowledge about humans is not possible without describing human experience as it is lived.*

An example of a question which could be explored through qualitative research would be: what are the attitudes of perioperative nurses towards patients who are HIV positive? These examples show the two major divisions of research. Each has a place in informing nursing practice.

Reviewing the literature

When a research question has been developed the next step is usually to search and review literature on the subject of the question. This establishes what is already known and not known about the subject, and can cause the question to be altered, refined or changed completely. Searching available literature may also reveal gaps and inconsistencies in current knowledge, perhaps providing further impetus for the research or influencing the way in which the research is carried out.

The purpose of the literature review is to obtain as comprehensive a view as possible of the subject of the research. The review is a 'critical summary of what is known about a particular topic' (Polit and Hungler, 1989). The way in which literature is used in the research study varies with the type of research and the design of research methods (Creswell, 1994). The importance of a literature search and review in any research project cannot be underestimated. Efficient and effective searching requires the development of skills which may have to be mastered before the research study can proceed. The rewards for this mastery will be realised in soundly based studies which are both academically and practically credible (Frank, 1996). Assignments for academic courses often use a review of the literature as an assessment task. For many nurses, this may be as close as they ever get to a research project. Using the opportunity to obtain and read a selection of literature on a subject related to practice can be a very rewarding and enlightening experience in itself.

Having retrieved the chosen literature, the researcher then has to analyse and evaluate it to illustrate accurately the subject matter. This may be difficult when little is known about a subject, or when what is known has not been widely published. In these cases, the researcher must look to related topics which influence and directly relate to the subject under study. This may mean evaluating research articles, and requires a critical and analytical examination which effectively dissects the work to reveal its strengths and weaknesses (Girden, 1996). This critical and questioning approach must be applied to all of the literature reviewed, whether research-based or not. Becoming the critical thinker which this demands stands any nurse in good stead for academic and research success.

Sampling

The sample of subjects selected to take part in the research must represent as closely as possible the whole of the population or group being studied. For instance, a sample of perioperative nurses should include full time, part time and night staff, as well as nurses working exclusively in particular areas (eg. anaesthetics, scrub, circulating and recovery). All clinical grades and ranks should be represented. For research targeted at one group or type of staff (eg. recovery), then the sample chosen should represent that group accurately in terms of grades, ranks, part time, full time.

Collecting data

The method or methods used to collect data will depend on the type of research being done and the type of data to be collected. Many types of data collection tools exist, some are specifically created for a particular study. Tools may be very simple, for instance a thermometer, or complex such as patient diaries recording their thoughts on illness and treatments. The choice of data collection methods, and whether these are already well established or created especially for the study are questions for the research student to answer and defend (Creswell, 1994). Specific collection tools may have to be designed and pilot studies carried out before the main study can proceed. This can be a tedious and frustrating time for the researcher, but may be time well spent as it adds to the credibility, reliability and validity of the study.

Researchers will be asked to demonstrate that their research is valid. Validity is the extent to which the research examines, measures or tests what it set out to examine, measure or test. In qualitative research, validity is defined as 'the extent to which the research findings represent reality' (Morse and Field, 1996). Reliability means the extent to which the research could be repeated and still produce the same or broadly similar results using another sample of the same population. It is quite permissible, and sometimes very useful, to replicate earlier research studies, as well as use other researchers' published tools and questions with your own sample. Copyright, correct references and acknowledgements must always be observed.

Data analysis

Analysing data transforms the raw facts, figures and text into an understandable form for presentation as findings of the study. It should provide the answer to the question: what does all this mean? This should also be the answer to the original research question, but may raise more questions than it answers. If this is the case, the research has not 'failed', it has increased the knowledge in a particular area and pointed the way to another question. Such is the enlargement and enrichment of knowledge.

Numerical data can be mathematically manipulated into statistics, tables, charts, graphs and the like, and will usually be done using a computer programme or programmes. Qualitative data in text form (eg. interview transcripts, questionnaires) can also be analysed by computer. The sheer volume and complexity of data can prove a daunting and overwhelming problem (Creswell, 1994), leading to the 'paralysis of analysis' syndrome. Research supervisors will advise on the best methods for data analysis, and these decisions should be made at the beginning of the study when the data collection tools are decided on.

Results

What the research study has found should be presented in an understandable form, clearly and accurately and, most importantly, without prejudice. At this stage it may become obvious that the answer which was sought has not been found, or that the research has revealed more questions than answers. This does not mean that the study was not worthwhile, or that it has no value. The results may reveal other important questions to be investigated, and other areas in need of research.

Honesty on the part of the researcher is essential. It is very tempting to look for and find what you so earnestly set out to seek. It may take courage to admit that the results may not be what was wanted or expected.

Evaluation and discussion of the findings

Whatever was revealed by the results has to be evaluated and discussed by the researcher. This process must be honest and open, as it will include a critical appraisal of what was done, what worked, what went wrong, and the overall implications of the study. After much hard work it may be apparent that what is required is more research. To what extent the results are applicable, and where and how they may be applied should also be evaluated. The researcher's interpretations and comments reveal how much has been learned from the study in terms of personal development as well as actual results (Greenfield, 1996). The university setting for nurse education now gives many more nurses the opportunity to become involved in research. Pre-registration programmes involve student nurses in finding, reading and analysing research throughout their training. Post basic education offers similar opportunities for qualified staff. In spite of this there is still far too little nursing research available to support practice. Nurses themselves can fill this gap, but knowledge applicable to nursing practice can also come from research into social sciences and psychology.

Quite apart from the difficulties of finding research on which to base practice, it is common to meet sustained opposition to changing practice once useful research has been found. Such opposition may be passive, where colleagues apparently accept information but make no attempt to put it into practice; or active, where despite proof, encouragement and effort, there is a refusal to change or even to sabotage new practices. It is very difficult to argue with a closed mind or minds. Such people hold back nurses and nursing, sometimes to the detriment of patient care.

Conclusion

Nursing will continue to struggle with its claim to professional status while practice is based on myths and traditions. Universities are the bedrock of research in other subjects, and are now available to nurses. The certainties of scientific studies used in medical research can be applied to some nursing problems, but qualitative methods have become equally acceptable and are the way forward for most nursing research (Morse and Field, 1996). Diploma, graduate and postgraduate studies are available in nursing and it is through these that nurses can establish the knowledge base which their practice needs.

References

Chapman H (1996) Why do nurses not make use of a solid research base? *Nurs Times* **92**(3): 38–39

Creswell J (1994) *Research Design: Qualitative and quantitative approaches*. Sage Publications, London

Dobrzykowski T (1994) Teaching strategies to promote critical thinking skills in nursing staff. *J Contin Ed Nurs* **25**(6): 272–276

Frank S (1996) Reviewing the literature: use of library and information systems. In: Greenfield T (ed) *Research Methods: Guidance for postgraduates*. Arnold, London

Girden E (1996) *Evaluating Research Articles From Start to Finish*. Sage Publications, London

Greenfield T (1996) *Research Methods Guidance for Postgraduates*. Arnold, London

Howenstein M, Bilodeau K, Brogna M, Good G (1996) Factors associated with critical thinking among nurses. *J Contin Ed Nurs* **27**(3): 100–103

Kitson A (1996) Editorial: Quality improvement, a multiprofessional commodity? *Qual in Health Care* **5**: 65–66

Mead D (1996) Using nursing initiatives to encourage the use of research. *Nurs Standard* **10**(19): 33–36.

Morse J, Field P (1996) *Nursing Research The application of qualitative approaches*. 2nd edn. Cheltenhan, Stanley Thornes

Polit D, Hungler B (1987) *Nursing Research Principles and Methods*. 3rd edn. Philadelphia, Lippincott.

Polit D, Hungler B (1989) *Essentials of Nursing Research*. 2nd edn. Philadelphia, Lippincott

Watson J (1981) Nursing's scientific quest. *Nurs Outlook* **29**(7): 413–416

8
Ethics and advocacy

Healthcare is the right of everyone. Disease is no respecter of people, colour, creed or social class. The professions which provide healthcare are ruled by ethically based codes of conduct based on morally acceptable behaviour (Smith *et al*, 1999). It is this basis of ethical responsibility which inspires the trust of patients in those who care for them. Knowing what is the right thing to do but not always being able to do it gives rise to ethical tensions in practice (Olson, 1998). Many ethical tensions arise from service expectations not being matched by resources. A survey of the readership of an American nursing journal (Ventura, 1999) revealed that these nurses were often dissatisfied with staffing levels: 'our readers told us they are short staffed on their units, and that this has had serious consequences... short staffing has put patients at risk and forced them to provide care with which they were not personally satisfied.' This situation will be only too familiar to perioperative nurses.

The UKCC *Code of Professional Conduct* (1992) expects nurses to defend patients by always acting in the best interests of those patients. Clearly, there are situations where there is a shortage of staff, inadequate care or where care is not in the patients' best interests, but sadly many nurses continue to work in such conditions for fear of the consequences of speaking out. Perhaps the best known British nurse who made a stand for better patient care was

Graham Pink. After being deserted by his nursing colleagues he was eventually disciplined and is no longer in nursing. Similar pressures and an acceptance of the inevitability of staff shortages is also reported in the American survey referred to earlier: 'Nearly 40% say they go to work and provide the best care they can under the circumstances.' Criticism is often seen as disloyalty (Haddad, 1999a).

Staff numbers are not the only resource in short supply. Inevitably, the cost of healthcare and the effect of this on the quality of care are also issues for nurses. Supplies, later admissions, premature discharges and increased surgical workloads are cited as being manipulated to allow maximum bed usage and throughput, 'patients are seen as dollar signs and not as people in need of help' (Wolfe, 1999). These may be the circumstances in which perioperative nurses may have to act as advocates for patients. Not all ethical decisions are concerned with the obvious shortages of staff and other resources described above. Here are three critical incidents from operating theatre practice where advocating for the patient was an issue.

The amputated toe

A very frail and ill gentleman was brought to theatre for the amputation of his right little toe. This was the information given on the operating list, and on the consent form signed by the patient. Due to the patient's poor state, the procedure was carried out using a spinal anaesthetic with sedation. When placed on the theatre table, the patient had dressings on both feet. The dressing on his right foot was wet with an offensive discharge. The dressing was removed to reveal a little toe that was black, and the other toes were a dusky bluish colour. The operation site was prepared and draped. The surgeon quickly amputated the little toe. While securing haemostasis in the wound, the surgeon took hold of the fourth toe, and immediately a large amount of pus and serous fluid oozed out from the base of the toe. It was obvious that the infection and necrosis extended well beyond the little toe. The surgeon looked carefully at the wound and the rest of the patient's foot. He asked the anaesthetist, 'Is he awake?' The anaesthetist replied, 'He's sedated'. The surgeon then stood by the patient's head, leaned down close to the patient's ear and called his name loudly. The patient made no response. The surgeon sat down and looked thoughtful. No-one spoke. The surgeon said to the scrub nurse, 'Give me the scalpel'. The nurse gave it to him. He held the patient's foot with his left hand and studied it carefully. He then gave the scalpel back to the nurse, completed the haemostasis and dressed the wound with the scrub nurse.

This patient needed an advocate to plead for his right to be consulted about further surgery. He had given his consent to the amputation of one toe only. It quickly became obvious that further surgery would be needed, and the surgeon may have been contemplating proceeding further at the time. No-one spoke on this patient's behalf. The surgeon decided for himself that it was not appropriate to proceed on this occasion. This begs the question of what should the scrub nurse or circulating nurse have done to advocate for this patient? Would they have felt empowered enough to challenge the surgeon if he had pursued further surgery for which consent had not been given? The ethical argument of beneficence is certainly applicable here. The surgeon, in extending the surgery would have undoubtedly been acting in the patient's best interests, but the situation was not life threatening and so there was time to inform and consult with the patient.

In this incident the principle of informed consent is the key issue. All too often the will of one person can be imposed on another who is not in a position to argue (Haddad, 1999b) and the potential for that was apparent in the incident. On questioning the surgeon about his decision after observing this incident, he said that he had contemplated extending the surgery, but decided that the patient would probably have to have the whole foot amputated. This needed to be explained to the patient and discussed with him.

The head injured patient

A theatre sister was about to go off duty when she was made aware that a patient with a head injury was having a CT scan and might need to come to theatre. She went to the scan department and looked at the films. She recognised the appearances of a blood clot on the surface of the brain, and saw that the patient was drowsy. She then overheard the registrar on the telephone to the consultant, reporting the scan findings to him. After finishing his conversation with the consultant, the registrar approached her and told her that he had sent for the anaesthetist and the patient would be coming to theatre. She asked,

'Is the consultant coming in?'

'No, he's told me to get on and do it' said the registrar.

'What are you going to do?' she asked.

'He needs a craniotomy' said the registrar, 'and I`ve not done one on my own before.'

The sister went back to theatre to prepare for the craniotomy. While waiting for the anaesthetist to arrive, the sister decided to telephone the consultant at home.

The following conversation ensued.

Sister: 'I hear you've asked the registrar to operate on this head injured patient.'

Consultant: 'Yes.'

Sister: 'Do you realise that he's not done a craniotomy without supervision before? He will take a lot longer than you would to open this patient's head, and the delay could affect the patient's outcome.'

Consultant: 'Well the patient's not too bad at the moment so I don't see what the worry is. I don't think the time factor is significant. Besides, you've helped with lots of craniotomies and can help him along.'

Sister: 'I'd really feel a lot happier if you'd come in at least to get the head opened.'

Consultant: 'I really don't see the need. The registrar will be fine, anyway, he will ring me again if there's any trouble.'

The patient came to theatre and the registrar operated with the assistance of a house officer and the theatre sister. The patient made a good recovery but was left with a slight deficit.

There is no way of knowing if the patient's outcome would have been different had the surgery been quicker. This patient had an advocate. The sister did plead on his behalf but to no avail. Being an advocate is never easy, though at least one can take comfort from having tried.

The action of contacting the consultant to express concerns about this episode is in keeping with the ethical principles of nursing (Ventura, 1999). The more difficult ethical questions arising from this incident concern the level of experience of the registrar, performing a procedure unsupervised for the first time. This was almost certainly never mentioned to the patient or his family.

Conflicting consent

A young man with learning difficulties was brought to theatre to have an inguinal hernia repaired. This young man had spent almost his entire life being cared for in hospitals and residential care, although his mother did maintain contact. His mother had signed the consent form, but the patient was accompanied to theatre by one of his regular carers. On checking the patient into theatre, the sister noticed that the consent form said, 'repair of left inguinal hernia', but the operating list for this patient said, 'repair of bilateral inguinal herniae'. On reporting this to the consultant, his reaction was that this poor man did have two hernias, but would be very upset by repeated surgery so it was better to do both at once, regardless of what was on the consent form.

The sister was not prepared to accept this and told the anaesthetist not to commence the anaesthetic until she had made an attempt to contact the man's mother. This produced an angry exchange between the anaesthetist and the sister, who were joined by the surgeon who asked, 'why can't we stop wasting time and just get on with this?'

Sister took the patient's notes and rang the contact number given for the man's mother. There was no reply. On reporting this to the surgeon and anaesthetist, the sister then asked, 'what are you going to do?'

The patient had a left inguinal hernia repaired. There is a conflict of interests here. The sister was indeed quite right to advocate for the patient to have only the surgery for which consent had been given, and to make the effort to contact his mother about the situation. On the other hand, she was exposing the patient to a further procedure which would be distressing for him. The question of this man's lack of ability to give his own consent meant that his advocate was pleading for him or his family to be given the same right to be consulted as any other patient. Knowing you are doing the right thing is not always a comfort.

The principle at stake here is autonomy, an individual's right to choose and act freely. This patient lacked the competence to make autonomous decisions, his mother had made the decision for him to have surgery on one hernia according to the form she had signed. Any proposed alteration to this should surely have been referred back to her unless the situation was life threatening — which in this case it was not. Perhaps the saddest reflection on this incident was that it might easily have been avoided, if the person who obtained consent from the patient's mother had ensured that the correct details were given and recorded on the consent form.

Conclusion

Obeying the law of the land is not difficult. In everyday life we do not even have to think about it. In perioperative nursing, only occasionally do questions of legality crop up. Ethics are another matter. When we encounter situations where our personal belief system or moral values are challenged, then the question of 'is this right?' becomes an issue. Advocating on behalf of a patient means exposing and perhaps justifying your own moral stance. This can be uncomfortable and leaves the individual open to challenge. The examples cited above were moral dilemmas for the nurses concerned, they had to decide at the time to speak out or stay silent and live with their consciences. This is the essence of ethics, you have to live with yourself and your actions or inactions.

References

Haddad A (1999a) Ethics in action [Acute Care Decisions]. *RN* **62**(1): 23–26

Haddad A (1999b) Ethics in Action [Acute Care Decisions]. *RN* **62**(3): 27–30

Olson L (1998) Hospital nurses' perceptions of the ethical climate of their work setting. *Image — J Nurs Scholarship* **30**(4): 345–349

Smith R, Hiatt H, Berwick D (1999) Shared ethical principles for everybody in health care. *Nurs Standard* **13**(19): 32–33

Ventura M (1999) Staffing Issues — Ethics on the job — a survey. *RN* **62**(2): 26–31

United Kingdom Central Council for Nursing, Midwifery and Health Visiting (1992) *The Code of Professional Conduct.* UKCC, London

Wolfe S (1999) Quality vs cost ethics on the job — a survey. *RN* **62**(1): 28–34

9
Organ donation

This subject raises questions which are closely related to the ethical discussions of the previous chapter. As organ transplantation is becoming increasingly common — it hardly ever makes the news these days — it will almost certainly become a part of perioperative practice for most nurses at some time in their career. There are many aspects of organ donation which remain controversial. In its earliest days a redefinition of death was required and, as the literature shows, even this fundamental question has still not been answered to the satisfaction of everyone.

Diagnosing brain stem death

In what proved to be a controversial editorial in the *BMJ*, Rodger Charlton stated that death was, 'a complete cessation of circulation to the normothermic adult brain for more than 10 minutes' which 'is incompatible with survival of brain tissue' (English, 1997). While most people would agree with this, correspondence in the *BMJ* following this editorial shows a disparity of views among the medical profession. English (1997) says that Charlton's view implies that periods of circulatory arrest shorter than ten minutes allow brain recovery, but points out that the accepted time for recoverable arrest is no longer than three minutes. Mardel (1997) reminds us that diagnosing death is not the important issue until resuscitation has been instigated, and followed by a thorough clinical examination. Mardel (1997) goes on to state that further dissection of the dying process by dividing it into 'somatic' and 'molecular' cloud the issue even further, and that death in his opinion is, 'the irreversible loss of capacity for consciousness, combined with the irreversible loss of the capacity to breathe (and hence sustain a spontaneous heartbeat)'. The medical royal colleges issued clearly defined criteria for the diagnosis of brain death in 1976.

These conflicting ideas do little to help nurses encountering organ donor patients in operating theatres. Burgoyne (1996) adds another dimension to the conflict, the impression given by the media that the decision to withdraw life support is taken by the patient's relatives. This is not usually the case as strict guidelines have to be observed and, 'there are legal requirements for the diagnosis of brain stem death involving two sets of tests performed by two senior doctors' (Burgoyne, 1996). Another point of contention is the time of death. Burgoyne (1996) says that it is after the second set of brain stem death tests. Others would argue that death occurs after the organs are removed, or when the ventilator is disconnected in theatre. It is difficult for theatre nurses to come to terms with the concept that the patient is already dead when they come to theatre warm, pink, with a heartbeat and respectable blood pressure. Patients for organ donation often arrive in theatre in better condition than trauma victims or patients with extensive disease.

Establishing brain stem death also means being absolutely sure that the patient's condition is not the result of metabolic failure, alcohol, or any kind of legal or illegal drug use. Patients who are admitted, resuscitated and then given relaxant drugs to enable ventilation must be very carefully assessed to ensure that their lack of spontaneous respiration and motor inertia is not the result of relaxant drugs or metabolic products.

The law would uphold the diagnosis of death of a qualified, experienced and practising doctor. This is relatively comforting, especially as it is usually a Senior Registrar or Consultant who would provide this. The Coroner has to be consulted in all cases of organ donation, and so the rigour applied to diagnosing death is subject to 'external' review by the Coroner who can refuse permission for organ donation where there is any doubt or where crime is suspected.

Heffernan (1998) provides an interesting and disturbing view of the legal aspects of organ donation in the United States, where laws vary from state to state. She cites a case where misinformation was given to a family who were approached to donate corneas and bone marrow. The family were assured that this could be accomplished without disfiguring the body. In fact, to obtain corneas both eyes are completely removed, and obtaining bone marrow involves removing the long bones from both legs — both highly disfiguring procedures. The family subsequently found out what had happened, sued the hospital and received an out of court settlement.

Informed consent and patients' rights

Before exploring consent, it is necessary to examine exactly what is meant by 'next of kin' as, in the case of organ donation, consent from the patient is not usually available. Donor cards, living wills and opt in or opt out systems will be covered later.

Caulfield *et al* (1998) ask if the term next of kin includes partners, including same sex partners, who are not related to the donor by blood or marriage? There are no clear answers to this question. Apparently there is no legal need for hospitals to have 'next of kin' included in patient documentation, nor is there any legal basis for nurses to assume that blood relatives have a different status or rights to partners in making health decisions for another adult (Caulfield *et al*, 1998). In reality, hospitals wish to cover themselves as far as possible against litigation and so try to ensure that they are able to contact an 'appropriate' person in case of sudden alteration in the condition of patients.

Donor cards, though carried by many people, have no legal standing where consent is concerned. They are an indication of the patient's wishes but are not enforceable without the consent of another person — usually the 'next of kin'. According to Raid and Banks (1990) 71% of people in the UK are in favour of organ donation, though only 23% carry donor cards. The position in Holland and Germany is similar. This is the 'opting in' system.

'Opting out', or 'presumed consent' which operates in Belgium and Austria, is the system where everyone is considered in agreement with donating their organs after death unless they have registered their decision to the contrary (Sells, 1990; Michielsen, 1992 cited by Gibson, 1996).

The American system of 'required request' means that relatives of all potential organ donors must be asked for the patient's organs by a member of the healthcare team (Norris cited by Gibson, 1996). A further complicating factor in the United States is the variation of laws between states. Malpere (1998) experienced the disturbing revelation that her husband's organs had been taken without her knowledge or consent in a state which practised 'presumed consent'. She is now calling for this law to be changed.

The situation in the United Kingdom is that 'the person lawfully in charge of the body may remove organs if having made such reasonable enquiry as is practical, that the deceased person or any surviving relatives has no objection' (Dimond, 1990 cited by Gibson, 1996).

Consent goes beyond legalities, and an examination of the ethics of organ donation is essential to any discussion. Moustarah (1998) sees this as a one-sided affair, declaring that 'it is ethically unacceptable to ignore the plight of patients who could be saved' in advocating for a policy of 'presumed consent' as practised in Belgium and Austria. This ignores the rights of the donor and the family involved. These rights are made explicit in The Department of Health (1998) campaign where they declare,

> *Organ donors must tell someone close to them because they are the people who will be asked for their agreement when the time comes.*

Organ donation reports, *Nursing Standard*, 1998

The importance of involving relatives after the death of a

loved one is graphically illustrated by Dix (1998) who lost her brother in the Lockerbie disaster and spent many years trying to come to terms with not being able to say goodbye to him.

For any form of consent to be valid in law, it must be seen to be 'informed'. Deciding to what extent the donor or the family are informed about what is involved in organ donation brings more uncomfortable questions but few answers. In the author's experience, very little or no information about the process of organ harvesting is offered or given to relatives. The potential recipient's plight is emphasised, and the positive aspects rightly highlighted. 'The ultimate gift' (Gibson, 1996) is an often quoted comforter, but the autonomy of potential donors may be ignored. Burgoyne (1996) assures readers of the very strict criteria which have to be followed, but this does not necessarily mean that informed consent is actually given.

The ubiquitous world wide web (www) now has a column in the *American Operating Room Nurses Journal* (AORN) and its first appearance was devoted to transplant information (Sjogren, 1998). This shows that information is widely available but nurses cannot assume what relatives and partners know. The debate regarding how informed is consent for organ donation will run and run.

Nurses' perceptions and experiences

An accusation sometimes levelled at nurses is that they resort to rituals to deal with uncomfortable or threatening situations (Walsh and Ford, 1989). Martin (1998) takes up this theme in relation to nurses acting as patient advocates. He declares that:

> *whilst maintaining an appearance of care, behaviour is structured to enable the nurse some degree of distancing.*

This author would argue that in order to cope with some aspects of organ donation, operating theatre nurses need to distance themselves to a certain extent.

Not all nurses are happy with the concept of brain stem death (Watkinson, 1995) and, as already discussed, the appearance of organ donor patients is not one of impending death. The need for research into nurses' experiences with organ donation has been identified (Watkinson, 1995), but such research when carried out may ignore theatre nurses as was the case with the study conducted by Pettier-Hibbert (1998).

Religion and belief may bring a crisis of conscience for the nurse. Nurses who practice certain faiths are allowed to withdraw from some surgical procedures which contradict that faith (eg. termination of pregnancy). There seems to be no clear-cut guidance for nurses where organ donation is involved.

There is a need for specialist nurse training for those involved with organ donation (Randhawa, 1998) but this seems to focus on ICU and other critical care nurses, with no mention of theatre staff. Is there an assumption here that the actual removal of the organs is not seen as traumatic for theatre staff; perhaps that it is just another type of surgery? Theatre nurses are isolated from the process of brain stem death testing and rarely meet the donor's family. This does not mean that they do not care.

Pettier-Hibbert's (1998) study of coping strategies used by nurses in dealing with organ donors and their families found that a number of strategies were apparent. One nurse's response after the diagnosis of brain stem death was, 'from then on, I don't think of them as a person because their personality, their temperament, and even their soul is gone... what makes them a person is gone and they're just a body now'. This is the organ donor that comes into theatre. Of the 17 nurses in Pettier-Hibbert's study, eight said that they continued to talk to the donor 'in case there was a little soul drifting' or that 'they still might be able to hear'. Remember these are ICU nurses, talking about the patient who will be cared for by theatre nurses. Fortunately in the light of these statements, Pettier-Hibbert recommends that dealing with crises, grief, ethics, morals, coping theories and spiritual issues be included in pre- and post-registration nurse education, and thankfully it is.

Conclusion

Organ donation is a significant contribution to health and function for patients who have no other hope of survival. It involves perioperative nurses in both the positive (receptor) and negative (donor) surgery. Death at any time evokes powerful emotions. For nurses dealing with otherwise fit people whose families have consented to the removal of organs for transplant, this is not 'normal' surgery. The emotions involved may be profound and disturbing, need to be acknowledged and dealt with sympathetically. Involvement at an earlier stage, and perhaps some shared care with ICU nurses, is a possible answer.

For nurses involved with patients who receive organs, the burden of the patients' expectations is immense. These patients are often close to death and fully aware that this is their only hope. Successful transplantation brings elation and joy, which may be short-lived. Failed transplants and intraoperative death may have to be dealt with too. This roller coaster of emotions can lead to burnout and stress for theatre nurses. Whatever involvement theatre nurses have with organ donors or recipients, such procedures can never be 'just another case'.

References

AORN Journal (1997) Speciality assembly members discuss their unique needs and interests at Congress meetings. *AORN* **66** (1): 70–71

Burgoyne T (1996) Strict watch. *Nurs Standard* **10**(45): 21

Caulfield H, Platzer H (1998) Next of kin. *Nurs Standard* **13**(7): 47–49

Department of Health (1998) *Code of Practice for the Diagnosis of Brain Stem Death*. HMSO, London

Dix P (1998) Access to the dead: the role of relatives in the aftermath of disaster *Lancet* **352**(133): 1061–1062

English T (1997) Diagnosing death: death of the brain stem means death of the patient. *Br Med J* **314**(7078): 443

Gibson V (1996) The factors influencing organ donation: a review of the literature. *J Adv Nurs* **23**(2) 353–356

Heffernan L (1998) Organ donation: the legal aspects. *RN* **61**(2): 51–54

Malpere H (1998) Organ donation isn't done by request only. *RN* **61**(4): 9

Mardel S (1997) Diagnosing death: start resuscitation first. *Br Med J* **314**(7078): 442

Martin G (1998) Ritual action and its effect on the role of the nurse as advocate. *J Adv Nurs* **27**(1): 189–194

Moustarah F (1998) Lets presume consent. *Can Med Assoc J* **158**(2): 231–234

Organ donation [reports] (1998) *Nurs Standard.* **13**(11) 33–34

Pettier-Hibbert M (1998) Coping strategies used by nurses to deal with the care of organ donors and their families. *Heart Lung: J Crit Acute Care* **27**(4): 230–237

Raid H, Banks R (1990) Recording patients views on organ donation: when to ask them and how to record the answer. *Br Med J* **301**(6744): 155

Randhawa G (1998) Specialist nurse training programme: dealing with asking for organ donation. *J Adv Nurs* **28**(2): 405–408

Sells S (1990) Organ commerce: ethics and expediency. *Transplant Proc* **22**(3): 93–932

Sjogren D (1998) Transplant information on the World Wide Web. *AORN J* **68**(6): 1035–1036

Walsh M, Ford P (1989) *Nursing Rituals: Research and rational actions*. Butterworth-Heinemann, London

Watkinson G (1995) A study of the perceptions and experiences of critical care nurses in caring for potential and actual organ donors: implications for nurse education. *J Adv Nurs* **22**(5): 929–940

10
Going to work and loving it...

There are as many ways of looking at the need to work as there are people doing it. For some, work is simply a means to an end, a way of making money, the necessary evil that pays for the things we need, and a myriad of other views. Most of the perioperative nurses the author has met regard their work as something more than a means to an end. They want to enjoy what they do, and enjoy themselves while they are doing it. To this end, many of the coping strategies used by perioperative nurses involve humour, and this is well supported in nursing literature. Hillman (1994) suggests that the interaction of nurses with high technology requires a, 'counterbalancing human response', and that humour and fun fulfil this role.

People use humour extensively as a form of communication (Sheldon, 1996), and it has been shown to have therapeutic value (Gilligan, 1993). Hillman's (1994) recognition of the effects of an increasingly technological approach to nursing was recognised by Sumners (1990) who observed how easy it might be to lose patients in the machinery which may surround them. Nowhere is this more appropriate than in perioperative settings. Sumners' study of nurse attitudes towards humour revealed largely positive attitudes towards using humour in a personal setting, but less positive attitudes towards using humour as a part of nursing care. Some of the respondents to the study revealed what many perioperative nurses say on a daily basis, 'I would go crazy if I didn't use humour'; 'If I didn't laugh in this setting I would cry'; 'In any practice setting involving people — humour is a must'.

Having fun at work has to be balanced by the need to observe proper professional behaviour towards patients, and always putting their needs before our own. The stressed and burned out nurse will be doing patients no favours if no safe outlet can be found for work induced stresses. Hillman (1994) reports that one of the first signs of burnout was the loss of a sense of humour at work. Being able to express happiness and joy are natural parts of everyday life, and so nurses need not feel guilty at including them in their working life (Mallet, 1993).

Humour can also be used as an aid to learning (Struthers, 1994), by linking facts to unlikely, bizarre, vulgar or sensual stems, students are more likely to remember them (Buzan, 1974). Teachers, however, need to exercise caution in the use of risqué references in lectures or handouts, as humour is a very personal construct and the potential for causing offence is always present. Harrison (1995) declares that the use of humour is indicative of a person's level of personal self-esteem and assertiveness. This is understandable as nurses in any learning situation would be reluctant to initiate a humorous exchange or remark if they did not feel it would be well received. The same author also points out that not all humour is kind and helpful, sarcasm can be particularly hurtful and has no place in a caring or educational setting. If humour is not a predominant feature in working or learning, most perioperative nurses realise the need for some kind of coping mechanism or strategy.

Nurses coping strategies were the subject of a study by Boey (1998). The findings revealed that the level of adaptation to the stresses of work was positively related to the level of job satisfaction. Nurses who coped with the stresses created by their jobs also reported that they were satisfied with their jobs. This bears out the author's experience of perioperative nurses, who either enjoy the role and its setting, or they do not. Perioperative nursing, and particularly work in operating theatres is something that you either like or hate. Very few nurses are ambivalent towards this type of nursing, and having chosen to work in it, then coping strategies are found or created. Boey's (1998) study found that nurses reporting high job satisfaction rarely resorted to defensive or avoidance coping mechanisms, indicating confident and positive approaches to work and personal psychological security. Working closely with consultant medical staff requires perioperative nurses to have these positive and confident approaches, and to feel personally secure.

The doctor-nurse game discussed earlier may contain some elements of humour, and certainly plays a part in job satisfaction and perceptions of self. Breaking a stressful and tense situation with appropriate conversation or a joke is often a psychological lifesaver, even if this entails one discipline gently 'sending up' the other one. Where the disciplines of medicine and nursing can develop a healthy symbiotic relationship, complementing each other's skills and enjoying mutual respect, both will benefit. Perioperative nursing offers many opportunities to develop such relationships, and to make everyone's working life easier. Hopefully, the contented work-force created by this will then deliver better quality care to patients.

Valuable though humour is there are other coping mechanisms which perioperative nurses resort to. Colleagues of the author tell of social gatherings as an important safety valve. Getting together away from work, even with people you see everyday, can lead to satisfying and supportive relationships which spill over into the workplace. Good friends can help get each other through stressful situations at home and at work. Even 'talking shop' in social situations can make light what was an apparent disaster a few hours before. Most of us can relate to feeling better after unloading the story of today into a sympathetic ear. If we can then bear to write all of our reflections down in a personal diary, mull them over at a later date and learn from them, we can begin to claim to be reflective practitioners and come to that 'positive sense of your own self worth' (Conway, 1996).

Nursing needs to celebrate successes, and prove their worth as a caring body. Redfern's and Noman's (1999) research showed that nurses valued effective, committed leadership and supportive colleagues. In spite of working in often impoverished conditions, good quality care is still most nurses' goal. Good quality care needs to be soundly based on research. Nurses are becoming research aware, they want to be a part of creating new knowledge and developing practice (Lipley, 1999). Clinical governance, and the audit process which informs it will take evidence from nursing practice as part of developing clinical excellence. Mary McClarey (1999), a non executive board member of the National Institute for Clinical Excellence (NICE) has already issued a call to nurses to send evidence of good practice to the board so that it may be recognised and shared.

The current emphasis on evidence-based practice is in

part at least driven by the academic preparation that nursing now has. Footit (1999) roundly condemns those who have questioned the university based training of nurses; I would urge those who feel like this to look at the advice of Mao Se Tung:

> *We think too small, like the frog at the bottom of the well. He thinks the sky is only as big as the top of the well. If he surfaced he would have an entirely different view.*

Gregory Dawes (1999) puts nursing knowledge, skill and competency into context:

> *The emerging value of competence needs to be recognised by perioperative nurses. The public expects safe and competent nursing care... we need to proudly show our patients that they can be confident that health care professionals remain competent years and decades after they have been in practice.*

Our former apprenticeship model of nurse training could never have delivered the confident, independent, critical thinking nurse produced and maintained by an evidence-based higher education programme. This author's nurse training, in a large teaching hospital thirty years ago produced nurses who were basically competent within a very limited range of practice, and who looked to the doctor for orders to be obeyed. Such reflections show just how far nursing has come.

The contribution nurses make to patient care is recognised by the current Government. The nursing strategy *Making a Difference* (DoH, 1999), published in July was warmly welcomed by nursing's representative bodies. The document sets out the Government's plans for the profession, and emphasises a commitment to recognising the value of nurses by putting in place a career structure which gives opportunities for improving clinical skills and creates new routes for progression (Lipley and Scott, 1999). Even if individuals take a pessimistic view of Government promises of progress for nursing, the fact that they have produced a strategy shows that they are at least acknowledging the importance of nurses to the health service and to patient care.

Perioperative nurses at all levels, regardless of their gender, need to accept responsibility and take control of their situation, as ownership and control are fundamental to managing change:

> *Freedom… involves rejecting the negative images of one's own culture and replacing them with pride and a sense of ability to function autonomously.*

> Roberts, 1983

There are many certainties in perioperative nursing, apart from death and taxes. There will never be a shortage of patients needing to be cared for. There is likely to be a shortage of perioperative nurses for the foreseeable future. Employment should be secure, with Trusts not wanting to waste skilled nurses. If you are genuinely discontented with your present situation then take the initiative and do something positive about it. Recognise your strengths and weaknesses. Capitalise on your strengths and start correcting your weaknesses. Invest in a professionally prepared curriculum vitae if a new job is your aim, but in any case, don't just sit there — do something. Apparently, 'the more you complain, the longer God lets you live' (source unknown — seen in a theatre changing room, where else!).

References

Boey K (1998) Coping and family relationships in stress resistance: a study of job satisfaction of nurses in Singapore. *Int J Nurs Stud* **35**(6): 353–356

Buzan T (1974) *Use your head*. British Broadcasting Corporation, London

Conway J (1996) *Nursing Expertise and Advanced Practice*. Quay Books, Mark Allen Publishing Limited, Dinton, Salisbury, Wiltshire

Department of Health (1999) *Making a Difference — A strategy for nursing in England*. HMSO, London

Footit B (1999) Leading nurses into the future. *Nurs Management* **6**(2): 23–26

Gilligan B (1993) A positive coping strategy. Humour in the oncology setting. *Prof Nurse* **8**(4) 231–233

Gregory Dawes B (1999) Skills, behaviours and motivation serve as a framework for competency. *AORN Journal* **70**(2): 188–190

Harrison N (1995) Using humour as an educational technique. *Prof Nurse* **11**(3): 198–199

Hillman S (1994) The healing power of humour at work. *Nurs Standard* **8**(42): 31–34

Lipley N (1999) Nurse practitioners will benefit from NICE plans. *Nurs Standard* **13**(29): 4

Lipley N, Scott G (1999) Professional bodies give unanimous support for Balir's nursing strategy. *Nurs Standard* **13**(43): 4–5

Mallet J (1993) Use of humour and laughter in patient care. *Br J Nurs* **2**(3): 172–175

McClarey M (1999) Its NICE to be recognised. *Nurs Standard* **13**(34): 26

Redfern S, Norman I (1999) Quality of nursing care as perceived by patients and their nurses: an application of the critical incident technique, Part 2. *J Adv Nurs* **8**(4): 414–421

Roberts S (1983) Oppressed group behaviour: implications for nursing. *Adv Nurs Sci* **5**(4): 21–30

Sheldon L (1996) An analysis of the impact of humour and its application to one aspect of children's nursing. *J Adv Nurs* **24**(6): 1175–1183

Sumners A (1990) Professional nurses' attitudes towards humour. *J Adv Nurs* **15**(2): 196–200

Struthers J (1994) An exploration into the role of humour in the nursing student — nurse teacher relationship. *J Adv Nurs* **19**(3): 486–491

Index